Germa

Organic germanium enha
enriches the body's oxygen supply, destroys toxic
free radicals, discharges heavy metals and other
poisons from the system and protects against
radiation. Here is the story of this newly available
trace element and what it can do for you.

'I think that Sandra Goodman is to be congratulated
for presenting clearly and concisely the information
so far available in an easily readable but scientific
way.' — *Dr Stephen Davies, Chairman of the British
Society for Nutritional Medicine.*

...ances the immune system,
...supply distribution...
...a healthy...
...best anti...
...the onu...

Germanium
The health and life enhancer

by

Sandra Goodman Ph.D.

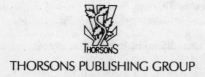

THORSONS PUBLISHING GROUP

First published 1988

© SANDRA GOODMAN 1988

British Library Cataloguing in Publication Data

Goodman, Sandra, 1951–
Germanium: the health and life enhancer.
1. Medicine. Drug Therapy. Germanium
I. Title
615'.315684

ISBN 0-7225-1633-9

Published by Thorsons Publishers Limited, Wellingborough, Northamptonshire, NN8 2RQ, England

Printed in Great Britain by Richard Clay Limited, Bungay, Suffolk

1 3 5 7 9 10 8 6 4 2

Contents

– Acknowledgements –

I am sincerely and deeply grateful for the initial inspiration and continued research support provided by the International Institute of Symbiotic Studies and for the ongoing symbiosis that has transpired between myself and Monica Bryant in giving birth to this work. I am also deeply appreciative to Steve Dalton for provision of a computer and to Andrew Collier for his continuing computer support throughout the completion of the various stages of this work. I thank Stephen Davies and Robert Erdmann for professional feedback and suggestions, and Sanum Kehlbeck and The Germanium Institute of North America for instructive materials. Also, with the sincerity of my heart, I thank the powers that be who have provided me with this most worthy task, and acknowledge the solidity of my parental upbringing, education and life experiences which enable me to be an instrument to advance the continuing work of integrating scientific knowledge with spiritual wisdom.

─── **Note to readers** ───

Before following the self-help advice given in this book readers are earnestly urged to give careful consideration to the nature of their particular health problem, and to consult a competent physician if in any doubt. This book should not be regarded as a substitute for professional medical treatment, and whilst every care is taken to ensure the accuracy of the content, the author and the publishers cannot accept legal responsibility for any problem arising out of the experimentation with the methods described.

Preface

You may never have heard of germanium before, except perhaps as a substance used for transistors. I hadn't until the day I was handed a plastic bag full of papers, a book on the subject, and asked to produce a summary report. Without preconceptions, or any burning interest in the subject, I started to read: the First International Conference on Germanium, Dr Asai's book, *Miracle Cure: Organic Germanium* literally hundreds of scientific papers and reports of natural practitioners, with extraordinary case studies.

I was turned on. As a scientist, I was impressed by the quality of the research, and the solidity of the documented data on germanium's therapeutic effects. Here is a substance which has been substantially researched medically, scientifically, and holistically for more than a decade, which has been elegantly documented as being non-toxic, immuno-enhancing, oxygen enriching, radiation and mutagenically protecting, detoxifying, as well as a potent analgesic. And this is merely a short list of germanium's attributes.

As an adventurous and curious individual who has partaken of the wisdom of various spiritual, esoteric and holistic practices on my own personal journey toward wholeness and well-being, I feel an extraordinary synchronicity about the task I have been given with this healing substance: to bring together the diverse sources of technical information about organic germanium into a readable and hopefully interesting form.

I am a scientific researcher. I am not involved in, nor do I have an interest in, sales, patents, or profits from germanium. I am, however, intensely fascinated by this trace element, and propelled by curiosity to discover unifying principles underlying germanium's ability to restore health to a diseased body. This element is the embodiment of an adaptogen, a holistic substance which restores balance to bodily functions, and I feel sincerely fortunate to have been handed the opportunity to review and disseminate information about its therapeutic properties.

Introduction

This book summarizes for the general reader the therapeutic properties of organic germanium, a health enhancing trace element. The information has been compiled from a broad spectrum of diverse sources, including medical and scientific journals, individual clinical practitioners, as well as case histories from the Asai germanium and European natural healing oriented clinics. It is astonishing and somewhat mystifying that a trace element with such a voluminous quantity of documented research has remained unrecognized before now by nutritionists and the medical profession. Apart from Dr Asai's own book, *Miracle Cure: Organic Germanium*, published in 1980, which has not been widely available, there is as yet no major consumer oriented book on the subject. In compiling this book, I am attempting to fill this gap.

Our understanding of the profoundly vital and therapeutic effects exerted by minerals has grown exponentially during the last few decades. Hard research data has documented the significant effects that minerals such as zinc, selenium, and chromium have on a multiplicity of conditions,[34,64,78,79] including immune function, heart disease, and blood sugar disorders. This has been reflected in the large number of books and articles appearing in health food stores, consumer magazines, and in the attention (and money) spent on nutritional supplementation. Minerals such as zinc, chromium, selenium, copper, manganese, molybdenum, and magnesium receive serious attention by medical and holistic practitioners alike.[15,40,112]

Organic germanium, not yet generally recognized as a nutritional supplement, will likely become a significant trace mineral because of its safety and versatile range of therapeutic properties, which have enabled somewhat 'miraculous' remissions and cures, particularly in the hands of the Japanese, who have had the most experience with this element. A critical analysis of the underlying mechanisms of how organic germanium works in performing its various tasks takes its effects out of the 'miraculous' and places them open to common sense understanding.

Germanium is not a magical substance, although its effects are sometimes remarkable. Germanium is a semi-metal which comes out of the earth and is present everywhere. Its elemental semiconductor properties made it highly prized by the electronics industry. Although it may not function analagously as a semiconductor in the body, organic germanium's electronic structure and configuration enable it to carry out many tasks which have a healing effect on the body, including the elimination and neutralization of toxic substances such as heavy metals and free radicals, and protection of blood cells from radiation. And elegant research at the molecular level has unambiguously documented organic germanium's immuno-enhancing properties, particularly in cancer and arthritis.

Organic germanium has been thoroughly researched by both the orthodox scientific and alternative holistic communities, with encouraging therapeutic results acceptable to the framework and philosophy of both these healing traditions. The versatility of organic germanium's therapeutic effects, and its virtual non-toxicity, make it a highly attractive substance to anyone interested in attaining and maintaining good health. I have been taking a nutritional (low) dose of organic germanium since I first encountered this work and I have felt that this substance has enhanced my energy level. I have also been impressed by the very positive, albeit anecdotal case history reports from clinics and practitioners all over the world. Therefore, based upon the extensive therapeutic and safety documentation on organic germanium, I would certainly encourage anyone to try it for him/herself.

Which brings the question full circle back to the individual, the most important component in the entire health equation. Organic germanium is not a 'magic bullet'. The individual is the healer, who, with judicious guidance and inner wisdom, chooses what works for him or her. Dr Asai believed that the most important criteria for getting better was the individual's conviction that he/she would get well. It has been scientifically established and accepted that our emotional state, stress level, and the food we eat all play an interrelated role in the function of our body's defence mechanism, the immune system, which to a large extent, determines our state of health. Nutrition, stress management, and preventive medicine are now indispensable tools of general medical practice. This book provides the most up-to-date information regarding organic germanium's many therapeutic properties.

—————— An overview of this book ——————

The initial chapters relate the intriguing history behind germanium, and describe the structure and therapeutic properties of the various organic compounds available.

The following chapters provide an in-depth report of organic germanium's health-enhancing properties: immune enhancement, oxygen enrichment, free radical scavenging, heavy metal detoxification, and radiation protection. This is followed by summaries of the research findings of organic germanium's action upon cancer, arthritis, senile osteoporosis, heart disease, mental illness, and other disorders.

The latter sections of this book discuss aspects of organic germanium vitally relevant to the potential consumer: safety, quality, sources, and therapeutic regimes.

The final chapters discuss esoteric and speculative aspects of organic germanium, concluding with a practical guide to holistic living, vibrant health, and individual fulfilment.

CHAPTER 1

Historical sketch: —— from element to —— organic compound

—————— Germanium the element ——————

Germanium as an element was identified in 1886 by a German chemist Clemens Winkler. The existence of an element with germanium's atomic structure was actually predicted by the Russian chemist Mendeleev, who left a space in his periodic table for an element which he named 'ekasilicon'. Winkler isolated this element during an analysis of the ore argyrodite, a silver mineral, from the Himmelsfurst mine, St Michaelis near Freiburg in Saxony, and named it germanium after his homeland. Germanium belongs to family four of the periodic table, along with carbon, silicon, tin, and lead, and is usually classified as a semi-metal, or said to have semiconductor properties.

Germanium is not that rare in the universe, with estimates ranging from 10 to 55 parts per million (ppm).[91] On the Earth's crust its concentration is approximately 6 ppm therefore it is more abundant than gold, silver, cadium, bismuth, antimony, and mercury, and in the same range as molybdenum, arsenic, tin, boron, and beryllium. Germanium rarely forms its own mineral deposits. In most cases, germanium is found in small (ppm) levels in the sulphidic ores of lead, zinc, and copper, although occasionally levels of 100 ppm have been found in deep thermal deposits of zinc. Germanium is highly concentrated in some coals, about 500 ppm. The highest reservoirs, world-wide, of germanium are found in Tsumeb (formerly German South West Africa) and Kipushi (Zaire), with concentrations reaching 1,000 ppm.

Technological applications of germanium

Several investigators studied microbial, medicinal and botanical effects of germanium during the 1920s and 30s, but until 1948, germanium was mainly relegated to the status of a rare element. Radar engineering prior to the Second World War had led to the use of crystal detectors based upon the use of germanium crystals, and in 1948 germanium was plucked from obscurity into the limelight by Bell Laboratories' researchers Brattain, Bardeen and Shockley, who utilized its semiconductor properties for the development of modern electronic devices, transistors and diodes.

During the seventies, germanium was replaced by silicon in the semiconductor engineering field; however, new areas of application opened up for this mineral. For germanium 'metal' these include: semiconductor photodiodes, rectifiers, and solar cells; special alloys for electronics and dental engineering; mirrors, optical systems, and radiation divisors for laser engineering; and infra-red engineering devices. Technological applications for germanium dioxide include the production of polyester chips, fluorescent tubes, special glass, and in the pharmaceutical industry, the production of therapeutically beneficial organic germanium compounds.

The birth of an idea:
———— Organic germanium as medicine ————

The events leading to the synthesis of an organic germanium compound with therapeutic properties are an inspiring tale, like many scientific discoveries, involving a mixture of serendipity, intuition, persistence, and faith. The figure of the now deceased Japanese researcher, Kazuhiko Asai, looms prominently in this story. For without Dr Asai's steadfast belief and ability to persist despite great personal hardship, it is hard to imagine how organic germanium could have made such a rapid leap from idea to actuality as a therapeutic compound.

Once something is created and exists in reality, it can be analysed, tested, and perhaps improved. However, the creative process, stemming from the conception of an idea and carried through to the birth of a tangible entity, is somewhat mysterious and awe-inspiring, which often provokes in the humble person gratitude to whatever forces inspired his insight. We owe tribute to discoverers like Asai, who make great sacrifices and commitments to follow their curiosity to completion. The story of Dr Asai's synthesis of the first organic germanium compound bears at least a brief telling. His book *Miracle Cure: Organic Germanium* is highly recommended.[2]

The connection between semiconductors and organic germanium is germane (no pun intended) to this saga, for Asai, upon reading about semiconductor properties of electrons of germanium, pondered over the effects such a substance might have in the body.

Germanium atomic number 32, has 32 electrons, four of which are constantly moving unsteadily along the outermost shell of the atom. These four electrons are negative electrical charge carriers and if approached by a foreign substance, one will be ejected out of its orbit. This famous phenomenon is known in electronics as the positive-hole effect which is so ingeniously utilized in forming transistors and diodes. When one of these four electrons is ejected, a positive- charge hole is created and the remaining three seize electrons from other atoms in order to maintain balance.[1]

Asai was specifically thinking about the process of dehydrogenation, and whether germanium might be effective in removing toxic hydrogen ions from the body. More about this later.

Research: germanium content in plants

In 1945 Asai helped to establish the Coal Research Foundation in Japan, from which came most of the early work on germanium. Research and painstaking analysis, in those days without sophisticated equipment, established the existence of germanium in Japanese coal, predominantly in the woody section, or vitrit. Asai intuited that the source of germanium in coal was from the plant matter, and not from the surrounding soil, which led to a whole series of experiments investigating germanium content in plants traditionally known to be therapeutic in Chinese medicine, such as shelf fungus, ginseng, Wisteria gall, and other health promoting foods including aloe, comfrey and garlic.[2]

Asai found high germanium content in these plants and hypothesized that germanium plays important roles in the photoelectrochemical process of photosynthesis, the metabolism and self-defence (protection from invading viruses) process of these plants. These questions regarding the role of germanium in plant metabolism and protection are undoubtedly important research topics for rigorous investigation.

At last, an organic germanium compound

Inorganic forms of germanium had been extracted from coal for use by the electronics industry. It now remained for Asai's group to do the reverse: convert the extracted inorganic germanium into an organic form. This turned out to be a laborious and daunting exercise which consumed more than a decade of painful, unfruitful failures. Concurrently, with the decline of the coal industry in Japan and Dr Asai's source of research funds, times were hard and Asai endured poverty with the exhaustion of his personal finances. Finally, a water-soluble organic germanium compound, carboxyethylgermanium sesquioxide, a white powder, was synthesized in November 1967. Asai, by this time suffering from severe rheumatoid arthritis, tested the germanium on his condition which, within ten days, had disappeared.

In *Miracle Cure: Organic Germanium,* [2] Asai condenses his more than 20 years of experience into a rather short volume, containing insights, hypotheses, and convictions, interspersed with experimental data. The incredible interest and research energy which has been expended over the decades is a testament to the courage, foresight and intuition of Dr Asai, for rigorous research has come far to date in documenting the scientific basis for Dr Asai's originally intuitive ideas of organic germanium's therapeutic properties.

CHAPTER 2

Organic germanium — compounds and — what they do

Twenty years have passed since the original synthesis of an organic germanium compound. During that period, organic germanium has been used clinically in many parts of the world to treat a wide spectrum of illnesses, and has been the subject of extensive research in many disciplines: pathology, biochemistry, pharmacology, immunology, oncology, and neurochemistry.

Organic germanium has been used in a broad spectrum of regimes: on its own, with diet and stress counselling, and as a drug in cancer trials, in conjunction with chemotherapy, radiation therapy, and surgery. Drawing these sources of information together gives quite a solid overview of the fundamental aspects of organic germanium.

The safety of organic germanium has been well-documented, as have its health-promoting effects in many diseases, including cancer and arthritis. Case histories, and in some instances clinical trials, have documented organic germanium's therapeutic effects in treating the following conditions:

Rheumatoid arthritis and rheumatism
Cancer: colon, prostate, breast, lung, ovarian, cervical
Leukemia
Asthma
Diabetes
Malaria
Senile osteoporosis
Mental disorders: depressive psychoses, schizophrenia
Pain

Digestive disorders: gastritis, ulcers

Influenza

Cardiac disorders: angina, hypertension, arteriosclerosis, apoplexy, cardiac infarction

Circulatory disturbances: Raynaud's disease

Parkinson's disease

Cerebral sclerosis

Skin eruptions: warts, corns, eczemas, burns, herpes

Epilepsy

Old-age infirmities

Amyloidosis

Myelo-optico-neuropathy

Eye diseases: glaucoma, black cataracts, detached retinas, inflammation of the retina and optic nerves, Behcet's disease

Double-blind, controlled studies have been carried out on several of the above conditions, particularly cancer. Although individual case histories are not in themselves sufficient proof to the scientist of a substance's effectiveness, positive results with organic germanium over many years with large numbers of patients and many disorders certainly provides a basis for more rigorous testing of organic germanium's therapeutic properties.

GE-132: Carboxyethylgermanium sesquioxide

The organic germanium compound carboxyethylgermanium sesquioxide (more accurately named mu-trioxo-bis [beta-carboxyethyl] germanic anhydride) or Ge-132 was synthesized by Asai's group in 1967. Details of its synthesis and crystal structure were published in 1976.[107]

The synthesis is carried out by the hydrolysis of an organogermanium trichloride. Of the four germanium electrons, three are bonded with an oxygen atom; the fourth electron is a free radical. A regular symmetrical lattice network is formed, as shown in Figure 1. The biochemical significance of this crystalline structure will become apparent in discussing organic germanium's ability to scavenge free radicals, protect against radiation, enrich the body's oxygen supply and rid the body of heavy metals.

Sanumgerman

Sanumgerman (chemical name: germanium-citrate-lactate) is an organic germanium product manufactured by Sanum–Kehlbeck in West Germany. This company has had a close association with Dr

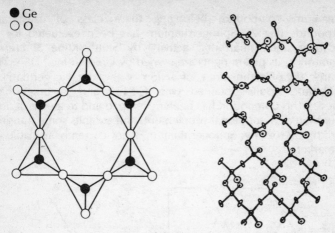

Figure 1

A beautiful geometrical pattern seen in the reticular structure of germanium
(From *Miracle Cure: Organic Germanium,* Japan Publications Inc.)

Asai, and has been developing and researching formulations of organic germanium for more than a decade.

The development of the organic germanium compound Sanumgerman grew out of the cancer research findings of oncologist Dr Seeger of the Robert -Koch Institute, Berlin, dating from 1938. Dr Seeger had been investigating electrochemical metabolic processes at the cellular level which caused normal cells to become cancerous. In his search for electronic acceptors which would cause cancer cells to revert to normal, he tested Dr Asai's organic germanium compound, which he found to be highly effective.

The close relationship between Dr Seeger and the research director of the firm Sanum–Kehlbeck, Heinrich Kehlbeck, deepened, with extensive research aimed at developing an effective organic germanium at Sanum's laboratories. After many years and variations of organic constituents, the compound germanium-lactate-citrate was found to be optimal.

Sanumgerman has been extensively used by health-care practitioners throughout Europe for about ten years. The safety and research data compare and confirm the results obtained with Ge-132, although no studies comparing the two formulations have as yet been done.

Spirogermanium

Spirogermanium, synthesized by Rice *et al.*[82], is an organic germanium compound, belonging to a class of azaspirane compounds (Fig 2). Spirogermanium has been evaluated for its anticancer and antiarthritic activity by Smith Kline & French Laboratories. Its patent rights are owned by Unimed Inc., USA. The research data on the mode of action of this organic germanium corroborate results obtained with Ge-132 and Sanumgerman; however, this compound has been developed and treated as a drug rather than as a nutritional supplement, and exhibits some transient neurological toxicity. Spirogermanium is not currently available on the market.

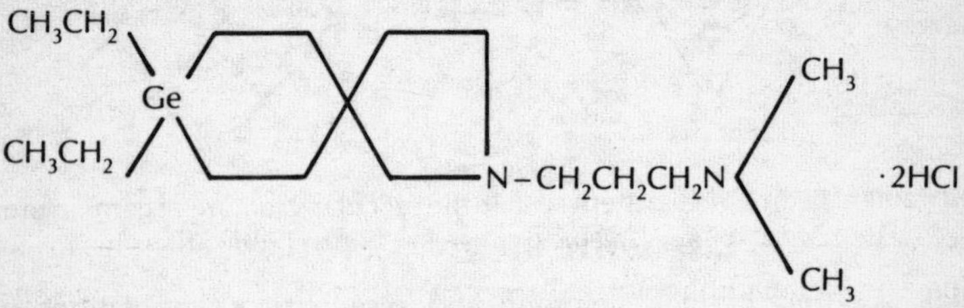

Figure 2
Spirogermanium

CHAPTER 3

Organic germanium — and the immune — system

Life without any defences

For a moment, imagine that you have been reduced in size to a microscopic speck of dust, and that you inhabit the world from this perspective. The air, which before had been a gentle, caressing breeze, now threatens to knock you over like a gale-force wind. Floating through the air, you are, in fact, a 'sitting duck' for bacteria, viruses, fungi, protozoans, and countless other miniscule creatures which you may have previously ignored or thoughtlessly trampled. You are seemingly naked and vulnerable to attack and engulfment. Pollutants, in the form of chemicals, acid rain, heavy metals, and radiation, natural and man-designed, all bombard you, and you are overwhelmed by the intensity of the onslaught. Your life is exceedingly short-lived.

This is not a dream or illusion. This is reality. We are, in fact, immersed in an atmosphere of potentially hostile chemicals and organisms which could literally wipe us out in short order. What prevents this from happening in the great majority of instances is our extraordinary defence network, the immune system. Even the word system does not do justice in conveying the intricately co-ordinated degree of orchestration that occurs between the many cells, organs and products of the immune system, which do such a masterful job of maintaining our biological, healthful integrity.

The media have reported about the tragically circumscribed lives of children born with deficient immune systems who need to live their lives in an artificial environment, a plastic sterilized bubble.

Heart transplant patients, who receive immunosuppressive drugs to minimize rejection, are kept in aseptic environments due to their susceptibility to opportunistic infections. And perhaps the most pervasive and generally life threatening of all immune diseases is AIDS (acquired immunodeficiency syndrome), associated with HIV (human immunodeficiency virus), which destroys key components of the immune system, leaving the person open to attack by organisms and infections that would normally be successfully countered by a properly functioning immune system. Contracting HIV, which destroys a key component necessary to initiate defence against infection, is tantamount to living naked without an immune system. However, as will be seen in this and other sections of the book, organic germanium is one of a variety of immuno-enhancing substances which can, by empowering the various components of the immune system, restore balance and thereby health to the individual.

Defence network—the germanium connection

The immune system is not simple. It is not just one organ, in one part of the body. It is an interconnected network of many types of specialized cells, primary and secondary organs, situated throughout the body, under hormonal control from the endocrine system, and open to modulation by the mind. Much scientifically detailed information has accumulated over recent years about the workings of the various components of the immune system. Our growing understanding of the interrelationship between the mind (thoughts), the emotions, the immune system and body health has come about partly as a result of research developments in the now interrelated fields of psychology, neurophysiology and biochemistry.[95]

Organic germanium is an immune modulator and enhancer. Elegant immunological research at the molecular level in Japan has elucidated the basis for organic germanium's antitumour activity. This has been found to be the co-ordinated interplay and expression of components of the immune system: interferon, macrophages, T suppressor cells and natural killer cells. There may be other immune components which may be modulated in other ways in other diseases, which have yet to be uncovered.

Germanium's immunomodulating properties are probably one of its most significant attributes, along with its oxygen enrichment and antioxidant properties, which explain its extraordinary effect in restoring health in so many types of illness. The immune system acts at a fundamental level of the body. Empowering the immune system is literally strengthening the basic building blocks or the foundation of a building. Strengthening the immune system will have far-reaching effects on every part of a person's body. Knowledge of the various cell types and overall functioning of the immune system may be critical to an individual, especially in view of the preponderance today of immune-type diseases, including cancer, AIDS, rheumatoid arthritis, and lupus erythematosa. An overall understanding of the immune system will enhance an individual's ability to assess the attributes of various immune modulating substances and to co-operate intelligently with the health practitioner.

———— Cells of the immune system ————

Just as organs are composed of various tissues, which are in turn composed of various cells, so the immune system is comprised of various tiers of organs and cell types, distributed all over the body. The main immune cell types are found among the so-called white cells, or leukocyte cells, which are distinct from red, oxygen carrying, cells of the blood. The main immune cells consist of B cells, T cells and macrophages. B and T cells, also called lymphocytes, begin life in the liver of a nine-week foetus, migrate to the bone marrow, where they begin to specialize, and develop along certain lines relating to their future function. The B cells (bone marrow derived) remain and mature in the bone marrow, while the T cells (thymus derived) migrate to the thymus gland where they mature.

One type of B cell is the plasma cell, which produces antibodies against foreign invaders called antigens. There are a number of antibodies, designated IgA, IgA, IgM, IgE, and IgD, which specialize in fighting different types of invaders of the body. Another type of B cell is the memory cell which helps to develop rapid antibody response to antigens to which the individual has previously been exposed. B cells are involved in humoral immunity.

There are various types of T cells, which, together with macrophages, are involved in cell-mediated immunity. These include T helper or T4 cells, which stimulate B cells and other T cells to activate an immune response to antigens. T4 cells are infected and destroyed by HIV. Because they are one of the first in a chain reaction of responses to infection, decimation of these cells by the AIDS virus leaves the individual vulnerable to attack from normally innocuous organisms. T suppressor or T8 cells, provide an immune feedback inhibitory mechanism, to keep the immune response in balance. T suppressor cells prevent B cells from being turned on by antigen, and inhibit T4 response. These cells have been found to inhibit expression of HIV in HIV seropositive men who are healthy and do not show symptoms of AIDS.[109] The induction of T suppressor cells by organic germanium is correlated with its antiarthritic activity. Other T cells are the natural killer or T cytotoxic cells which combat foreign cells directly with toxin. Macrophages are produced in the bone marrow. They surround and gobble up antigens (a process known as phagocytosis) , processing them for easier recognition by T cells.

One class of substances produced by white cells, and which plays a vital role in the whole interplay of immune cell types, is the interferons, which possess potent antiviral acticity. As we shall see, organic germanium stimulates the production of interferon which plays a key role in immune modulation and anticancer activity.

——— Organs of the immune system ———

The primary organs of the immune or lymphatic system are the thymus and bone marrow. The thymus gland, pyramid shaped with many lobes, each with an outer cortex and an inner medulla, is located beneath the breastbone. The T cells mature in the cortex, then migrate to the medulla for release during immune challenge. The bone marrow, site of red cell and macrophage production, and B cell maturation, is the soft material found in the long bones of the arms and legs.

One of the secondary organs of the immune system is actually a network of lymph nodes, situated throughout the body and interconnected via vessels which drain the organs served. Lymph nodes are compartmentalized with B cells, T cells and macrophages. The spleen, located on the left side of the abdomen between the stomach, kidney, and ribs facilitates the interaction of B cells, T cells, macrophages and antigen-reactive cells, and aids in the recirculation of white cells. Another secondary organ, the tonsils, also contains B and T cells. The other secondary immune organs are the appendix, Peyer's patches, and intestinal nodes, which serve as drainage points of the lymphatic system. They are also the site of B cell maturation and antibody production in the intestines.

Organic germanium's immuno-enhancing ——————— properties ———————

Elegant research at the molecular and clinical levels has reproducibly demonstrated that organic germanium has significant immuno-enhancing properties in animals and humans. Furthermore, the mechanism of organic germanium's antitumour activity has been proposed as the co-ordinated modulation of immune components. The following is a list of organic germanium's known actions on the immune system; it is indeed possible that organic germanium influences other immune transmitters that remain to be investigated.

1. Organic germanium stimulates the production of immune (gamma) interferon.
2. Organic germanium activates resting macrophages and converts them to cytoxic (killer) macrophages.
3. Organic germanium stimulates natural killer (NK) cell activity.
4. Organic germanium stimulates the production of T suppressor cells.
5. Organic germanium augments decreased immunity and restores impaired immunoresponse in aged mice.

The detailed published research studies which document the above statements are fully cited at the end of the book.[3,4,71,86,98-103,105] Many of these have been carried out by Japanese researchers with Ge-132. However, reports of Sanumgerman's augmentation of natural killer cells and Spirogermanium's induction of T suppressor cells would seem to indicate that all these organic germanium compounds are immuno-modulatory in similar fundamental ways.

Organic germanium induces interferon with anti-viral activity

United States Patent No. 4,473,581, entitled 'Organogermanium Induction of Interferon Production',[43] describes in detail immune properties of Ge-132, in particular those related to the production of interferon. These are summarized below:

1. The antiviral activity, or ability of the induced interferon to inhibit viral replication was investigated. Viral infection inhibitory activity, which was dose dependent and species specific, was detected in the serum of mice 25 hours after administration of Ge-132.
2. From the physical and chemical analyses, it was concluded that the interferon induced was immune (type II) gamma interferon.
3. Ge-132 induced the formation of activated macrophages in mice cells.
4. Ge-induced interferon displays marked antitumour activity, through the activity of activated macrophages.
5. Ge induces interferon and activated macrophages in humans as well as in mice.

Organic germanium enhances activity of natural killer (NK) cells

1. Administration of Sanumgerman to mice significantly enhanced the cytolytic activity of natural killer (NK) cells, in a dose-response manner.[30]
2. These stimulatory effects were seen as early as day 2, peaked at about day 4, and by days 6–8 returned to normal.
3. Compared to controls of 10 per cent cytolysis, the activity of NK cells of germanium-treated mice reached 27–33 per cent cytolysis.

Antitumour activity of organic germanium via immune modulation

The unravelling of how organic germanium works in inhibiting cancer growth, as it reads in the published literature, is like an exciting mystery novel. I would like to summarize one small example from this scientific saga, without intending to slight the many other contributors along the way. The researchers are Suzuki, Brutkiewicz and Pollard, collaborating scientists from Japan and the USA. Up until then, the following was known:

1. Ge-132 exhibited antitumour activity against certain cancerous tumours.
2. T cells and macrophages were involved in anticancer protection.
3. The protective effect could be transferred to tumour-bearing mice either by Ge-sera (interferon) or Ge-macrophages.
4. Macrophages from Ge-treated mice could inhibit tumour growth *in vitro*.
5. Interferon was present in Ge-treated mice. When the interferon was inactivated, the antitumour activity was abolished.

The foregoing suggested that T cells, macrophages and lymphokine(s), or interferon, all played a role in the expression of the antitumour effect of Ge-132. The scientists then set about determining the co-operative role of the macrophages and the lymphokine (or interferon) in Ge-132's antitumour activity. The results of these experiments were published in 1986.[103] The sequence by which organic germanium inhibits tumour growth is via the following coordinated immune modulations:

1. Ge stimulates T cells to produce circulatory lymphokines (most likely gamma interferon).
2. These lymphokines (interferon) generate activated macrophages from resting macrophages.

3. The tumours are inhibited by the activated macrophages.

The conclusions drawn from this work illustrate the fine detail in understanding that has evolved from research on the immunological modulations effected by organic germanium. Further fine details are added here, but it is almost certain that research has far outstripped the published literature from 1986.

1. Ge requires T cells to produce its antitumour effects, but T cells themselves are not required in the host for the antitumour effect. It is suggested that Ge needs T cells to produce the gamma interferon, which plays a role in antitumour activity.
2. Ge activates macrophages, antitumour activity of Ge is expressed in conjunction with macrophage functions, and Ge requires activated macrophages for expression of antitumour activity.

Relationship of the immune system to the entire organism

When focusing on the fine microscopic details of scientific research, one frequently cannot see 'the forest for the trees'. The individual components of the immune system, the T cells, natural killer cells, macrophages, etc., are the tools by which we are healed. There is an organic process, encompassing the mind, emitting thoughts and emotions, involving the food and chemicals we ingest, our genetic makeup, our general physical condition, all of which activate various neurotransmitters and immunotransmitters which then travel to the various organs and call into effect the 'foot soldiers', the immune cells, which actually attack and destroy the foreign invaders.

Organic germanium, with its potent immunostimulatory effects, can be a powerful healer, especially when supported by other health-supporting practices, such as mental relaxation, proper nutrition, and exercise. These facts should be especially borne in mind with respect to the most challenging and pervasive disease of the immune system—AIDS.

———— Organic germanium and AIDS? ————

In AIDS, HIV infects and destroys T4 or T helper cells, which are the cells which help to turn on the entire immune response process.[27,28] The gradual result of this is an almost total immune vulnerability of the individual to any foreign antigen. There are several approaches to AIDS:

1. Develop a vaccine which stimulates the production of antibodies

which kill the virus, thereby conferring immunity on the individual.

2. Apply substances which either prevent HIV from infecting T4 cells, such as AL-721, the alternative 'active lipids' treatment, or inhibit its replication, like AZT, the orthodox drug.

3. Work with the body's own immuno-enhancing mechanisms of keeping the virus in check, such as T suppressor cells, which appear to prevent the expression of the virus, as reported by researchers in California in 1986.[75,109]

4. Strengthen the immune system using all means available: meditation, stress reduction, diet, nutrition, exercise, emotional and spiritual fulfilment.

All of these strategies are valuable, and should be pursued concurrently. The bulk of research money is currently devoted to the development of a vaccine, and the majority of media coverage ignores other treatments which may be less spectacular, but in the end may save lives without adverse side-effects or huge sums of money. It would appear to make good scientific as well as common sense that, by strengthening all aspects of the immune system, an individual with HIV infection could manage to keep healthy and prevent the development of AIDS. Publications detailing results of various alternative treatments of HIV infection are appended at the end of this book.[5,112]

There is no scientific literature published to date regarding the effects of organic germanium on AIDS or on HIV. However, in view of organic germanium's effects on stimulating interferon, enchancing natural killer cell activity, and activating macrophages and T suppressor cells, it would appear eminently plausible that organic germanium could have invaluable therapeutic properties in the treatment of AIDS, without any of the toxic side-effects accompanying so many of the present drug treatments. Germanium was discussed as a potentially promising anti-AIDS agent at a conference held in Japan in 1987.[92]

Several preliminary anecdotal case reports have been communicated about the successful use of organic germanium in clearing Kaposi's sarcoma and other lesions. With a view to establishing scientifically the possible therapeutic value of organic germanium, and to stimulating interest in organic germanium AIDS research, the author is presently planning a double-blind trial using organic germanium with AIDS patients in the UK.

The immune system is not an isolated part of the body—it is

integrally linked to the whole organism, and is therefore amenable to enhancement by many practices. Organic germanium appears to enhance and restore balance at a fundamental level and therefore supports health in a thoroughly natural way.

CHAPTER 4

Organic germanium: —— oxygen enricher —— and antioxidant

—————— Oxygen—the vital link ——————

Oxygen — breath of life, prana, universal life energy, and fuel. Without oxygen we die. Pollution of the atmosphere with toxic chemicals, degradation of the ozone layer by fluorocarbons, destruction of the tropical rain forests with its plethora of life forms, all ultimately affect that which we breathe in which fuels life. In addition to food, raw materials, splendour, and spiritual enrichment derived from the many forms of plant life, our lives depend on our green co-inhabitors of this planet for oxygen which is evolved from photosynthesis.

A person can live for perhaps months without food, perhaps several days to a week without water, but within three to five minutes of stopping breathing, irreversible damage occurs to brain cells. Many health-enhancing practices are centred around increasing our supply of oxygen. Aerobic exercise is known to benefit the immune system as well as the heart; hence today's emphasis on fitness, in activities ranging from walking and swimming to dancing and running. The breath is used in meditation practices as a means of focusing one's concentration, in rebirthing to help people relive and more positively integrate experiences which they may have blocked from consciousness. Breathing deeply is an effective way of easing pain and fear, and in certain clinical practices, hyperbaric oxygenation is used therapeutically to increase the body's oxygen supply. Life saving emergency procedures of resuscitation stress the importance of starting and maintaining a person's breathing, and hence their oxygen connection. From the most ancient to the most modern practices, the breath and oxygen perform vital roles.

Oxygen is a vital as well as a precious substance; oxygen supports our life; it is the substance which is required to drive our cellular metabolism. Cells deprived of oxygen simply cannot sustain normal metabolic functions. A condition known as hypoxia (low oxygen) invites cellular vulnerability which may lead to cellular degeneration, ageing and cancer. Our primary mode of metabolism is oxygen driven. The nutrients we ingest are digested via biochemical pathways, in which complex molecules are broken down into simpler substances, and energy is generated and stored as molecules of adenosine triphosphate (ATP). Oxygen is required to fuel this process. If there is not an adequate supply of oxygen, non-oxygen (anaerobic) biochemical pathways go into operation. An anaerobic environment in our bodies encourages the proliferation of pathogenic microflora, such as candida; it also supports cancer cells, which are thought to revert to an anaerobic form of metabolism.

Oxygen is literally a life-sustaining substance to our bodies. A few of the oxygen-requiring processes that are constantly going on are: digestion and absorption of nutrients we ingest; detoxification of poisonous substances we inhale from the air we breathe, ingest in the food we ear, and absorb from toxic heavy metals such as mercury which are placed in our mouths as dental fillings. When we stress our bodies, through consumption of caffeine, excess sugar, meat, alcohol, drugs, lack of sleep, mental and emotional pressure, oxygen is needed to repair the damage done to our cells, tissues, and organs. The immune system requires oxygen to protect the body from foreign attack; the phagocytic white cells which engulf and destroy foreign invaders, actually 'zap' their targets with a dose of toxic superoxide.[62,63]

—— Reactive oxygen toxic species (ROTS) ——

For all of oxygen's vital, life-giving properties, there is also a negative side: this is in the form of certain toxic oxygen species generated during the metabolic process, which are extremely reactive and are now thought to be the primary cause of cellular degeneration, ageing and many diseases including cancer. These reactive oxygen toxic species (ROTS) include superoxide, hydrogen peroxide, hydroxyl radical, and singlet oxygen. These oxygen species are toxic because they have acquired an extra electron which makes them extremely unstable. They are 'free radicals', are incomplete by themselves, and are extremely reactive and damaging to cells. (Hydrogen peroxide is not, strictly speaking a free radical, but is an incompletely reduced form of molecular oxygen.) A more comprehensive discussion of ROTS and their role in many diseases is outlined in an elegant and articulate book by Bradford *et al* entitled *Oxidology*.[10]

The body has managed to put some of these ROTS to practical uses in bodily processes, for example the use of superoxide by phagocytes to kill their target cells as mentioned above. The body also has developed natural ways of neutralizing or destroying these ROTS; substances which can detoxify ROTS are called antioxidants, free radical scavengers, or oxidative scavengers. For example, a natural antioxidant of superoxide is superoxide dismutase (SOD); catalase and glutathione (GSH) are antioxidants of hydrogen peroxide. Certain nutrients, including vitamins C and E, are dietary antioxidants of hydroxyl radical and singlet oxygen respectively, while the trace mineral selenium is an antioxidant of hydrogen peroxide, through its intimate association with the glutathione enzyme system.

Organic germanium—oxygen enricher and antioxidant

Organic germanium enriches the body's oxygen supply and is also a potent antioxidant, properties which contribute to this trace element's widespread beneficial effects upon many interrelated metabolic process in the body.[62,63] Although organic germanium's properties of oxygen modulation are not yet precisely elucidated, there is sufficient clinical research evidence to lay the goundwork for more detailed cellular investigation.

Organic germanium enriches oxygen supply

1. Organic germanium lowers the requirement for oxygen consumption by organs in culture and increases the life span of animals under oxygen stress.

Experiments, conducted with mice in a biochemical laboratory of Tohoku University, investigating the effects of organic germanium upon oxygen consumption in the liver and diaphragm indicated a decline in oxygen consumption. Dr Asai has postulated that organic germanium plays the same role as oxygen in the body, thereby increasing the body's oxygen supply. There is a relationship between oxygen supply, blood viscosity and blood flow. When more oxygen is available, blood viscosity decreases, thereby increasing blood flow to all organs.

2. Organic germanium protects against carbon monoxide

asphyxiation, stroke, and Raynaud's disease, conditions linked with oxygen starvation.

Upon taking therapeutic doses of organic germanium, there is often a warm, glowing, even a tingling, feeling that has been attributed by Dr Asai to its oxygenation effect. Individuals suffering from diseases of the circulatory system, such as Raynaud's disease, which may lead to gangrene and limb amputation, have shown significant improvement to their condition after taking organic germanium.

3. Organic germanium is beneficial in treating eye diseases and wounds, especially burns.

Organic germanium has been successfully used to treat various eye diseases, including glaucoma, black cataracts, detached retinas, retinal inflammation, and burns. It is not yet known which therapeutic properties of organic germanium effected these improvements; however, it is a reasonable supposition that the oxygenation effects of organic germanium contributed to the healing of these conditions.

4. Organic germanium, in conjunction with hyperbaric oxygen treatment,[65] can bring about significant improvement in cases of multiple sclerosis and other degenerative conditions.

The naturopath Jan de Vries writes about the beneficial effects of increased oxygenation in treating cases of multiple sclerosis in his book *By Appointment Only*.[18] De Vries actually met Dr Asai in 1975[17] and has been using organic germanium in his practice. He is currently compiling many of his case histories of germanium treatment in cancer and leukemia, to include in a book. He writes: 'hyperbaric oxygen treatment, in combination with germanium, can improve the condition of a patient beyond belief...Eyesight often improves when a multiple sclerosis patient has hyperbaric oxygen treatment, because good eyesight depends on a good supply of oxygen in the blood.'

5. The structure of organic germanium, a crystalline lattice network extensively bonded with negative oxygen ions, is said to actually substitute for oxygen, and to enable the attraction and elimination of acidifying hydrogen ions, which detoxifies the blood.

In the electron transport scheme during oxidative metabolism, electrons are transferred along a set of electron acceptors, and, with the combination of hydrogen and oxygen, ultimately form water. However, when there is an oxygen deficiency , the loss of electrons can result in the accumulation of positive hydrogen ions, which lead to blood acidification. Ge-132 has negatively charged oxygen ions, which can clear away these hydrogen ions and thus detoxify the blood.

6. Organic germanium's ability to easily transfer electrons permits it to act as an electron sink during oxidative metabolism, thus enhancing the body's generation of energy without the intake of extra oxygen.

The electron transport system can be likened to a fire bucket brigade. If there is a shortage of electron acceptors, the entire process can grind to a halt, just as if one person is not in position, the bucket of water cannot get passed to put out the fire. Organic germanium has been shown to be an excellent electron conductor, and thus can significantly contribute to the efficiency of the entire process of oxidative metabolism, which ultimately generates energy for the body.

Organic germanium is an antioxidant

1. Organic germanium (Ge-132) protects against the accumulation of amyloid, a free-radical oxidative end-product, in mice.[97]

A disease called amyloidosis results from an imbalance in the process of protein breakdown, resulting in the accumulation of amyloid. Amyloidosis may be associated with chronic inflammatory diseases, immune amyloidosis with plasma cell disorders, localized amyloid deposition in neuroendocrine organs, or congenital deficiency of enzymes which break down amyloid precursors. Reports in the clinical literature report that amyloidosis can be induced by immunosuppressive agents. In a laboratory study in Japan, organic germanium significantly inhibited (50 per cent of the untreated group) the induction of amyloidosis in mice. The mechanisms of this suppression remain to be elucidated.

2. Organic germanium (Ge-132) protects cysteine, a sulphhydryl amino acid, from becoming oxidized in solution.[104]

Cysteine is a sulphur-containing amino acid. Solutions of cysteine have been found to have favourable effects upon eye conditions, notably corneal ulcers and burns. However, water solutions of cysteine are rather rapidly oxidized to form an insoluble product, necessitating the constant preparation of new solutions. Germanium was found to stabilize solutions of cysteine and inhibit its oxidation; preparations remained water soluble for up to one week. This demonstates one therapeutic application of germanium's antioxidant properties.

3. Organic germanium (Sanumgerman) has significant activating effects upon superoxide dismutase (SOD) and glutathione-related enzyme systems in rats.[37] The dose-related dynamics of activation are different for the two enzyme systems.

Several doctoral dissertations from the Institute of Physiological Chemistry in Hanover[23] deal with the effects of organic germanium compounds (Sanumgerman and variants of the formulation) upon glutathione-related enzyme systems as well as superoxide dismutase in rats. These results are consolidated here:

(a) Cytoplasmic and microsomal glutathione-S-transferase were activated.
(b) Glutathione peroxidases (GSH-Px) were activated, the concentration of reduced glutathione (GSH) increased, whereas total glutathione (TG) levels were affected according to the particular organic ligand of germanium used.
(c) Activation of superoxide dismutase (SOD) activity was biphasic, dose-dependent, as well as affected by the particular type of germanium organic ligand used.
(d) Catalase activity of liver mitochondria and peroxisomes is modulated according to dose and germanium substance used.

The ability or organic germanium to modulate the activities of known antioxidants glutathione (GSH), superoxide dismutase (SOD) and possibly catalase, provides solid evidence of organic germanium's antioxidant properties.

—————— Can structure be the key? ——————

Central to organic germanium's oxidizing and antioxidant properties is its structure, which, as noted in Chapter 2, is a crystalline lattice network, extensively oxygen bonded (Fig 3). Germanium has four electrons, three of which, in Ge-132, are bonded to oxygen, the other being a free radical able to interact in diverse reactions, which has implications for properties in addition to oxygen modulating, including protection from radiation and analgesia. Sanumgerman (germanium citrate lactate), has a different structure, but similar oxygen-enriching properties and rigorously documented antioxidant effects. Therefore, it may be this electronic facility which enables organic germanium to give and take so freely, electronically speaking, which is central to its oxygenation and antioxidant properties.

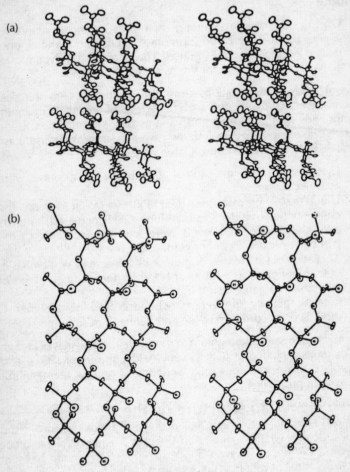

Figure 3

(a) A stereoview of a portion of the carboxyethylgermanium sesquioxide lattice array.

(b) A stereoview showing the layer network of carboxyethylgermanium sesquioxide and the atomic numbering scheme.

(From the Journal of the American Chemical Society, 8 December 1976.)

CHAPTER 5

Protection from —— heavy metal and —— radiation poisoning

—————— **The hazards of being alive today** ——————

The least expected, and hence the most insidious, dangers to life come on silent wings—in the air we breathe, the water we drink and the food we eat. When we are in a car crash or explosion, at least we know where the broken limbs or burns were sustained. However, silent deadly killers like heavy metals (mercury, lead, cadmium) and radiation (atmospheric fall-out, industrial waste, medical and dental procedures), exert a cumulative toxicity upon living organisms.

Thanks to considerable pressure exerted by environmental groups upon governmental bodies, there has been a growing awareness in all sectors of society of the dangers to life and health caused by heavy metal and radioactive contamination. The pollutants are myriad in number: carcinogenic organic chemicals, acid rain causing fuel stacks, teratogenic (causing deformities to embryos) chemicals in the plastics industry, leaching of phosphates from fertilizer application, lead from automobile exhausts, mercury in fish and algae, radioactive fall-out from Chernobyl, to name but a very few.

The industrial workplace can be exceedingly hazardous in many occupations: coal and asbestos mining, chemistry laboratories, dental practices, and nuclear medicine departments. Awareness of the dangers of these substances has led to greater safety precautions: the wearing of gas masks, lead aprons, clinical monitoring of blood and urine. However, it would be naïve to think that we can escape these silent but lethal poisons anywhere on this industrialized planet. Simply being alive and breathing, we are inevitably exposed to numerous toxic substances.

The dangers of heavy metal poisoning

One of the most lethal poisons known is mercury, which is put into our mouths as dental amalgam for fillings[96,118] and is found in common household products, such as thermometers and batteries. Some of the toxic effects caused by mercury poisoning include headaches, limb tremors, tingling, depression, heart and other organ problems, which sometimes appear decades after exposure to the poisonous substance. Lead, is also a lethal poison ever-present in paints, pipes, automobile and industrial exhausts, has been insinuated as a factor in the decline of the Roman Empire, and more recently as a source of poisoning of slaves and slave owners in sugar plantations in the Caribbean. Cadmium, also found in batteries, is yet another toxic heavy metal. Heavy metals, such as mercury, lead and cadmium, are not easily discharged from the body—they linger and accumulate while exerting their toxic effects.

No safe limit of radiation

The threat posed to our very existence by radiation is widely known and reported; fear of nuclear war is considered to be a major factor in the psychological profile of a significant number of young people alive today. Yet, leaving aside the gross dangers posed by threat of nuclear war, or the melt down of a nuclear power plant, there are still the exposures that result from simply living in today's world—atmospheric fall-out, medical and dental procedures, and industrial uses of radioactive products, such as the irradiation of food to prolong its shelf life.[111]

Recently, a programme aired on British television documented the radioactive contamination of drinking water in the South-east, including London region, by a manufacturer of radioactive isotopes for medical and research purposes. Once radioactivity, or any other poison, gets into the atmosphere, the water, or the earth, it enters the food chain and affects a myriad of organisms, including microbes, insects, plant life, animals, and humans. Radioactivity decays; however, some isotopes have half-lives of hundreds of years or longer, contaminating a site for many generations.

There have been standards established by the International Commission on Radiological Protection (ICRP) of a so-called 'acceptable' dose of radiation exposure. In 1957 this was set at 5 rem per year for a worker or 0.5 rem for a member of the general public. Also, dose levels for each organ of the body have been established. Since that time, it has been realized that this is an unacceptable level of risk, and that 'acceptable' doses should be below 1 rem. These risk levels have been calculated on a probability that 1 in 10,000 workers will die each year, or that over a lifetime 1 in 200 workers will die from an radiation-related accident at work. These risks do not take into account non-fatal damage such as cancer, damage to developing foetuses, and the general debilitating effects of exposure to radiation. It is generally accepted working premise by most informed researchers that there is no risk-free dose of radiation; we just may not be able to quantify the damage which occurs over an extended period of exposure to radiation.[111]

Awareness and personal commitment

To maintain optimum health it is necessary to minimize, as far as is practically possible, our exposure to industrial toxins and atmospheric pollutants, by carefully choosing where we live, refusing to permit aerial spraying of toxic substances such as insecticides, the building of polluting power-generating stations, and by taking measures which enhance the body's natural mechanisms for dealing with poisons—the immune system, antioxidants and other natural detoxifiers found in various herbs, seaweeds and minerals.[16]

Japan—natural choice for mercury and radiation research

Organic germanium was first developed and tested in Japan, where the first atomic bomb was exploded at Hiroshima, and where thousands of people suffered the hideous effects of a disease called Minamata disease caused by eating fish poisoned with mercury. Out of the horrors and misery of radiation and mercury poisoning has come awareness and, hopefully, more alertness to the consequences of our actions upon our environment. For example, when I was a graduate student the best methods available for analysing the structure of nucleic acids was electrophoresis with methyl mercury. Because of the known toxicity of methyl mercury, and indeed, most of the other chemicals we were using, great attention was paid to safety measures to prevent exposure to such substances. However, great vigilance is required to safeguard our health. It was because of the shocking reports from the Minamata sufferers in the Japanese population that Dr Asai undertook some research into organic germanium's effects upon mercury in the body.

Organic germanium captures and discharges mercury [2]

In one experiment, mercury chloride was intravenously injected into a rat and induced the formation of a calcareous deposit in the cortex and medulla regions of the kidney. After 10 days' treatment with organic germanium, most of the calcareous deposits had disappeared, and within a further 20 days, no trace of calcium could be observed. Dead cells were found to be dispersed, in the tissue interstices. After 30 days of organic germanium treatment, the dead cells had been replaced by healthy cells.

Another experiment, again in rats, described how the administration of organic germanium at the same time as mercury protected against the development of any toxic symptoms, thus apparently preventing mercury poisoning.

Similar types of experiments were also performed using cadmium, another heavy metal toxin, which indicated that organic germanium could discharge this poison from the body.

How organic germanium discharges heavy metals

The toxicity from mercury is thought to arise from the interaction of mercury with free organic radicals, causing electromagnetic disturbances, affecting cells and organs possibly quite distant from the point of entry.[96] The most effective way of avoiding mercury poisoning is to prevent its accumulation through discharging. Dr Asai has theorized how organic germanium may accomplish this—again, through the unique structure of this molecule (Fig 4).

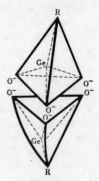

Figure 4

The cubic structure of the organic germanium compound showing three negative oxygen ions around germanium.

(From *Miracle Cure: Organic Germanium,* Japan Publications Inc.)

The organic germanium compound has a cubic structure with three negative oxygen ions around germanium. The negative oxygen ions are at the base of the cubic triangle. Two cubic triangles whose bases face each other make a molecule. (See diagram). Any heavy metal accumulated in a living body is in a state of positive ions which would jump into and be trapped in the mesh structure of the negatively-charged oxygen ions of the organic germanium compound taken into the body.[2]

This would explain organic germanium's apparently beneficial effect of 'capturing' other heavy metals, such as cadmium. Although there are no published data on Sanumgerman or Spirogermanium's application in this regard, since they also have lattice structures extensively oxygen bonded, it could be predicted they would act in a similar way. Other trace minerals such as selenium have been shown to enhance the discharge of heavy metals; however, the mechanisms may be quite distinct. This is certainly an area open to research, not only for mercury, but for lead, cadmium, and other toxic heavy metals.

Organic germanium: antimutagen against ─────── radiation and chemicals ───────

Japanese researchers Kada *et al.* have published the results of microbial genetic research documenting germanium's potent ability to protect bacterial cells from mutation due to gamma irradiation and to a known chemical mutagen Trp-P-2 (3-amino-1-methyl-5H-pyrido(4.3-b)indole). In carefully controlled experiments subject to rigorous controls, Ge-132 was shown to reduce mutations in *E coli* due to gamma radiation by twentyfold.[72] In a discussion of the possible mechanisms for this antimutagenicity, it was suggested that Ge-132 may improve the fidelity, during DNA synthesis, of DNA polymerase III, a DNA-replicating enzyme. This has been shown to be the case with cobaltous antimutagen. Germanium oxide was shown to reduce the mutation rate in *Salmonella typhimurium* induced by Trp-P-2, by 40–67 fold.[44] The mechanism for this mutation protection was also suggested to occur through amplifying the fidelity of DNA repair systems of the cell, not resident on a plasmid (extrachromosomal DNA).

These experiments at the molecular level offer solid evidence of organic and inorganic germanium's ability to significantly protect against genetic mutations from gamma radiation and a known chemical mutagen.

Organic germanium protects against radiation damage in humans

The administration of Spirogermanium to rats induces the production of radiation resistant (2,000 rad) T suppressor cells, as described in Chapter 8. Administration of organic germanium to patients undergoing radiation therapy for cancer offers protection against radiation-induced killing of white and red blood cells. What is needed most to fight cancer is a strong immune system; chemotherapy and radiation therapy are often toxic to 'normal' and cancerous cells alike, thereby wiping out the white cells of the immune system, leaving the patient extremely vulnerable to infection. The ability to irradiate and kill cancer cells while leaving the immune system intact would offer a significant advantage to any cancer patient, and would provide a magnificent example of using holistic and allopathic medicine in a complementary manner for the optimum health of the patient.

The following case history illustrating the radiation-protecting effects of organic germanium is summarized from Dr Asai's book:[2]

The patient, male, age not disclosed, had suffered amputation of the lower left leg, due to a cartilage tumour in the left heel. Several years later, due to the development of a cartilagenous tumour in the right lung, a lobectomy of the middle and lower lobes of the lung was performed. However, a thumb-sized tumour had started to develop in the remaining portion of the lung.

The man then started to avail himself of various natural medicine therapies—herbs, cold and hot stimulation therapy, Demiger therapy, fasting, phototherapy, finger-pressure therapy, electric vibrator, and a strict macrobiotic diet. He then tried ozone therapy, acupuncture, and vacuum blood purification therapy, but the tumour continued to grow.

At this point the man began taking organic germanium—120 ml liquid solution and 200 mg powder per day. At the advice of the doctors at the germanium clinic, cobalt radiation to kill the malignant cells was initiated. A large dose of 1,000 mg organic germanium was administered to reduce the damaging effects of the radiation.

During 47 almost consecutive daily colbalt radiation treatments, the man's physical strength and growing appetite was sustained. There was hardly any change to the blood data as is shown in the table [see page 45].

During the angiographic examination, the man experienced no pain, in sharp contrast to an agonizing experience two years earlier. A tumour, weighing about 2 kg was removed. Following the operation, the man's appearance was much improved upon from the previous surgery. He began to eat solid foods on the third day, to walk on the fourth. The stitches were removed on the tenth day and he returned home on the eighteenth day. He then returned to field work as a farmer.

Blood data before and after cobalt radiation

	Start	After 47th radiation
White blood cells	3,100	3,000
Red blood cells	507	513
Blood platelets	10.2	9.6
T.P.	7.4	7.4
A/G	1.5	1.55
GOT	37	35
GPT	28	30

How does organic germanium protect against radiation damage?

The precise mechanisms describing how organic germanium can protect human cells from radiation damage have not been elucidated. However, Dr Asai referred to data indicating that 'atoms of organic germanium securely fasten to red blood cells and shelter the cells from oncoming electrons by diverting them around the atom'.

In the absence of further data, one could postulate various means by which organic germanium could have an affinity for blood cells, possibly by electronic attraction. And given germanium's extended network shape and its ability to conduct electrons efficiently, the foregoing certainly appears to be a reasonable possibility.

The above data definitely indicate the lack of destruction of blood cells following a course of cobalt radiation treatment. These data, in conjunction with the Spirogermanium data of the generation of radiation resistant T cells, offer evidence of the protective effect of organic germanium—this certainly could be further investigated.

CHAPTER 6

Neurotransmitter
——— modulation ———
and analgesia

Psychoneuroimmunology—
——— the mind/body link ———

A profoundly fertile interdisciplinary field of research probes the intimate connections that exist between the mind, the brain, the nervous system and the immune system. The phrase that describes the interaction of the central nervous system and the immune system is 'psychoneuroimmunology'.[95] Whereas Western science's previously simplistic and mechanistic world view of matter, including the body, would dissect and describe each individual organ, tissue, and cell and ascribe a specific cause and effect to it, it has become obvious that the chemicals in the body, and the body systems, are interrelated. And, although the interactions of the mind, the nervous system and the immune system cannot be termed simple, the emerging complexity interweaves with a rather elegant holism, in which simple molecules are modulators and effectors in both the nervous and the immune system.

Pain perception and response

This interrelation of the mind, the body and the immune system is fascinatingly embodied in the phenomenon of pain perception and response. In a simple example, pain is a warning signal conveyed from cells at the site of injury via nerves to the brain. More complex is the phenomenon of phantom limb pain, in which pain apparently emanates from an amputated limb. The gate theory, proposed by pain expert Ronald Melzack, suggests that there is a certain threshold of pain, influenced by a variety of neurophysiological and psychological factors.

Thus, how strongly the pain is felt, and what physical and emotional responses are evoked, are determined by a myriad of parameters, ranging from the context of the situation, our psychological state, and our general physical and mental fitness. In life-threatening situations, such as in war, natural disasters such as floods or earthquakes, or traumatic catastrophes, such as mine disasters, nuclear accidents, or hostage incidents, individuals have been known to become endowed with an almost 'superhuman' degree of strength, courage, and a seeming lack of pain until well after the events when they can afford the luxury of being in pain. There have been many inspiring tales of victims trapped for extended periods of time in seemingly hopeless situations, who have virtually willed their way to survival. The body seems to focus attention on the most life-threatening stimulus—a headache seems to fade when one is knocked on the head.

Our response to pain can be modified by our moods—somehow, pain feels worse when we are depressed, hopeless, alone, and unloved. When we are happy, fulfilled, and free from stress, even severe pain can be accepted with equanimity and not lead to a downward spiralling of emotional depression. Pain can be modulated by a variety of mechanisms, including simply distracting the focus of attention and becoming absorbed in something else, by altered states of consciousness achieved through breathing, exercise, meditation, and hypnosis.

—— Components of the nervous system ——

The nervous system is a massive network which reaches to almost every part of the body. Within different sites of the brain are control sites for many body functions. The cortex, the outer 'grey matter', is the site where vision, hearing, and calculations occur. Deeper into the brain is the limbic lobe, site of emotions, such as anger, fear, love, joy, and stress. Still deeper is the hypothalamus, the interface between the brain and many peripheral regulatory functions. The hypothalamus regulates many of the body's automatic or autonomic functions which continue whether we are awake or sleeping, such as breathing, digestion, and heartbeat. The hypothalamus, highly concentrated with neurotransmitters, communication molecules of the nervous system, also sends neurohormones to the pituitary, which is the body's master gland, which, in response to messages received by the hypothalamus, sends hormones to specific organs throughout the body.

Chemical messengers of the nervous system

There are various molecules which act as messengers to facilitate the transmission of information throughout the body. These are termed neuroendocrines, neurotransmitters and neuropeptides. Amino acids, in addition to being the building blocks of protein, are also the precursors to small molecules which modulate the nervous system by acting as neurotransmitters. For example acetylcholine, which stimulates nervous system function and also immune functions, is a general transmitter between neurons, including nerve endings of skeletal muscle fibres.

A group of neurotransmitting molecules, collectively called catecholamines, includes dopamine, noradrenaline, and adrenalin. Deficiencies in dopamine have been noted in Parkinson's disease, leading to muscular tremors. Yet another neurotransmitter is serotonin, which is an inhibitory neurotransmitter involved in cognitive functions and sleep cycles. Paradoxically, although serotonin exerts calming effects on the nervous system, it is overall an immunosuppressant. Another group of molecules called neuropeptides include the opioid (morphine-like) peptides beta-endorphins, and enkephalins. These peptides, which appear to be the body's natural pain-relieving molecules, are released by the hypothalamus in response to pain, and can profoundly modulate reactions of the nervous system. Although their immune effects are not yet completely known, it has been shown that beta-endorphins increase T-cell proliferation and enkephalins enhance active T-cell rosettes.[5]

—— Organic germanium's effect upon pain ——

One of the most widely appearing 'anecdotal' reports in case histories of patients treated either in Dr Asai's Germanium Clinic, or with European physicians, is the alleviation of pain with the administration of organic germanium. This includes terminal cancer victims, sufferers of arthritis, and angina patients. Dr Asai himself described the virtual absence of pain and the improved sense of well-being associated with cancer surgery after taking large doses of organic germanium. One man with a cartilagenous tumour of the lung underwent an angiogram, which previously had been excruciating, without pain.

Since pain is also subjectively modulated by mood, belief, hope, stress, etc., these reports of lessening of pain might be attributed to psychological factors rather than organic germanium. However, recent neuropharmacological data attained through laboratory animal studies, has demonstrated concrete results attesting to organic germanium's neuromodulatory and analgesic properties.

Organic germanium's modulation of neurotransmitters

The effect of Sanumgerman upon the central nervous system in mice has been investigated,[50,51] and has been found to influence both the catecholaminergic and the serotoninergic systems. Sanumgerman reduces levels of noradrenaline and dopamine and inhibits their utilization in the brains of mice, while stimulating serotonin and serotonin-turnover rates. Therefore, overall, Sanumgerman has been found to exert an inhibitory effect upon the catecholaminergic system and a stimulatory effect upon the serotoninergic central system. These actions would explain some of the transient side-effects sometimes seen with Spirogermanium, such as lethargy, drowsiness, and defective vision. The stimulation of serotonin, which exerts a calming effect, can explain the positive effects of feeling better which are consistently observed with patients taking organic germanium.

Organic germanium's analgesic effect via neuropeptides

Ge-132, administered to rats orally or by intraperitoneal injection, enhanced the effects of morphine analgesia;[36] the analgesic action was completely blocked by naloxone, which is a stereospecific opiate antagonist. This suggests that Ge-132 may activate the analgesic system through an opioid receptor in the brain, activate dopaminergic or serotoninergic neurons in the analgesic pathway operated by morphine, and release endogenous enkephalins or other neuropeptides.

Further elucidation of organic germanium's analgesic effects by Komuro *et al.*[55] showed that derivatives of Ge-132 inhibited the degradation of endogenous opioid peptides (enkephalin-degrading enzymes). In this report, 28 species of Ge-132 derivatives were examined for their inhibitory effects on these enkephalin-degrading enzymes, purified from a number of animal and human organs and tissues. Several derivatives inhibited the activity of dipeptidyl-carboxypeptidase from longitudinal muscle tissue, aminopeptidase from human cerebrospinal fluid, and dipeptidylaminopeptidase from monkey brain and bovine small intestine longitudinal muscle. This evidence strongly suggests that organic germanium's analgesic effect comes about through preventing the degradation of enkephalins, one of the body's natural class of pain-relieving molecules.

CHAPTER 7

Germanium's —— action against —— cancer

——— Cancer—a philosophical treatise ———

We must go back to basics to answer the question 'What is cancer?'. We are so conditioned to going into a state of shock at the very mention of the word that we hardly think rationally of just what cancer is. It is, stated very simply, the uncontrolled proliferation of cells. Normally, our immune system can handle foreign cells, toxins, and abnormal, cancerous cells. However, due to a multiplicity of factors, perhaps genetic predisposition, poor diet, toxic environmental attack, recreational abuse, negativity, and depression, our 'resistance' weakens, abnormal cells multiply and start to spread, somehow oblivious to normal control mechanisms.

Nowhere is the split between allopathic and holistic medicine more pronounced than in diseases such as cancer. Western science, stuck in the notion 'one disease, one cause', spends billions of dollars in many highly focused races to find a cure for a 'disease' of a body. Hench the 'search and destroy' methodology of chemotherapy, radiation therapy, radical surgery, all in the sincere desire that to be healed, the cancer must be destroyed.

A holistic approach to healing considers all factors of the individual: psychological/spiritual, emotional, environmental, as well as physical. Where is the cancer? What in that person's life has caused him to create a cancer in that part of the body? What is the physical and genetic disposition of the person, his parents? What has been his diet? How stressful is his work? Is he fulfilled emotionally and spiritually? Does he exercise?

Diagnosis and treatment of cancer would ideally utilize, in a co-operative fashion, the most appropriate techniques of modern medicine and/or complementary therapies, with the patient playing an active role in his treatment and healing.[9] This type of treatment would use to maximum advantage technological advances of modern medicine as well as the accumulated wisdom of traditional healing practices.

The approaches used with germanium in the East and West exemplify almost perfectly the dichotomy between the two healing traditions. On the one hand, the Asai Germanium Clinic prescribes organic germanium, along with a non-acid forming diet and stress counselling for its cancer patients. At the other extreme, North American oncology groups administer Spirogermanium in intra-venous drips to cancer patients[116] who have already undergone every other option before being admitted to the germanium clinical trial.

Chapter 13 compares and evaluates in detail, the philosophy and practice of each of these approaches, as well as those taking a middle line. This chapter summarizes the scientific research which documents organic germanium as a therapeutic agent in cancer treatment.

—— Germanium—cancer research studies ——

There are normally several distinct stages whereby a potential cancer drug is tested before it can be made available. If the substance demonstrates anticancer activity in a number of assays *in vitro* (in the test tube), then studies on animals will be conducted. If these studies demonstrate promising results, then experiments and trials will be conducted with actual human cancer patients. Because organic germanium is a natural substance with virtually no demonstrated toxicity (see Chapter 11 on safety), germanium is classified as a food supplement and not a drug, which has enabled faster progress in establishing its therapeutic action in humans for many serious illnesses, including cancer. Thus, treatment of human cancer patients over almost two decades has occurred in parallel with the careful scientific studies in animals, establishing its anticancer action, resulting in a wealth of documentation from the human side, as well as laboratory data. There are business and philosophical issues deriving from this question of 'Food or drug?' which will be addressed in Chapter 12.

Putting together the cancer research studies of the three organic germanium compounds, Ge-132, Sanumgerman and Spirogermanium, at the cellular level, in animals and human cancer patients, the evidence for organic germanium's anticancer properties is solid and reproducible. This chapter will highlight the research results in these various areas.

Cellular level

1. The allium test uses actively dividing plant cells to measure the anticancer or oncostatic activity of a potential anticancer substance. Sanumgerman, when analyzed by this procedure, showed the characteristics of an active compound.[35,53,61]

2. Tests with various laboratory cancerous cell lines demonstrated that Spirogermanium inhibited DNA, RNA and protein synthesis of these cancer cells at very low concentrations.[87,117]

3. Further characterization of organic germanium's mode of action at the cellular and molecular level, showed that germanium compounds inhibited viral (HSV-1) replication *in vitro* and blocked the synthesis of DNA in hepatoma 22A and ovarian cancer cells.[38,39,67]

Animal studies

1. Sanumgerman's antitumour activity with several types of cancers has been documented in mice. In one study, the group of mice which received Sanumgerman had a 20 per cent incidence of tumours, compared to 50 per cent in the control group.[13] Also, Sanumgerman administered to mice with carcinoma of the colon survived longer.[60] In other studies, Sanumgerman showed positive results against colon, lung and myeloma type cancers.[59]

2. In studies with rats, Spirogermanium was shown to increase the lifespan by 500 per cent of animals with Walker type carcinoma.[114]

3. Ge-132 has shown significant antitumour activity against a wide spectrum of tumours,[52,57,70,100] which has been elegantly shown to be mediated by activation of immune mechanisms, including macrophages, natural killer cells, interferon, and T suppressor cells (see also Chapter 3).

The above-cited animal studies with organic germanium compounds were conducted by a variety of established scientific groups around the world, in accordance with scientifically accepted protocols, such as those set down by the National Cancer Institute, USA. The results have been published in learned refereed scientific journals, attesting to the fact that the methodology and data analysis were subjected to controls associated with scientific methodology. Although this in itself is no guarantee of a substance's efficacy in humans, it does attest to the fact that organic germanium compounds demonstrate significant anticancer activity in laboratory animals infected with a wide range of different cancers.

——————— Human cancer patients ———————

Clinical trials

1. Clinical trials on lung cancer showed a statistically significant effect of Ge-132 upon life prolongation, tumour regression and overall improvement in performance status and immunological parameters. A double-blind controlled study for unresectable lung cancer was commenced in 1980.[70] The patients were divided into classes, depending on the type of cancer. The treatments consisted either of chemotherapy plus Ge-132, or chemotherapy plus a placebo, administered double-blind, meaning that neither the patient nor the doctor knew whether the individual was receiving germanium or the placebo. Interim results to date revealed a significant difference between the placebo and Ge-132 in the proportion of partial and complete responses to treatment with organic germanium.

2. A technical document issued by the Asai Germanium Research Institute, compiles clinical and research data on the pharmacological, immunological, and toxicological properties of Ge-132.[29] The long list of studies, trials and investigators in the Appendix attests to the intense research activity ongoing in Japan, to 'evaluate strictly the therapeutic efficacy of Ge-132'.

3. A clinical study of Sanumgerman's effectiveness against ovarian malignancy was conducted with six women, aged 44–64, who had been operated for malignant tumours of the ovaries and uterus.[84] The well-being of all these patients improved noticeably, and they experienced considerable relief from pain. The remarkable analgesic (pain-relieving) properties of organic germanium are reviewed in Chapter 6. In five out of the six women, there was no exudate formation in the abdominal or inner pelvic cavity; a slight exudate was observed in the sixth woman.

4. A phase I clinical trial was conducted with 35 patients with a variety of cancers, with intravenously administered Spirogermanium.[87,88] This trial was conducted in order to define a tolerated dosage and to determine anticancer activity. Several of the patients experienced mild transient side-effects such as dizziness which were all resolved within a few minutes to several

hours. There was no evidence of cumulative toxicity, nor of bone marrow depression. One patient showed a partial response in the palpable lymph nodes for two months.

5. A phase II trial for patients with lymphoma-proliferative disease (non-Hodgkin's lymphoma and Hodgkin's disease) was conducted with Spirogermanium. Out of 17 patients, 5 (30 per cent) demonstrated an objective response, including two complete responses. No haematological toxicity was observed.[87]

Excerpted case histories

1. Reduction in the size of a splenic tumour was achieved after three week's Sanumgerman, orally administered to a 62-year-old woman with myeloproliferate syndrome.[54]

2. An 18-year-old male with embryonal cancer of the testicles and lung filae, undergoing a variety of therapeutic regimes, including Sanumgerman, recovered, with no metastases up to the present (1985).[84]

3. A 55-year-old woman who had been operated on for sigmacarcinoma, developed metastases in the stomach, kidney, mesenterium, and liver. Following cytostatic (chemo) therapy, she received Sanumgerman treatment. Dark-field analysis of her red blood picture was closely monitored. After three months of treatment with Sanumgerman, there was a significant decrease in erythrombic development, with considerable improvement in cell respiration. Four years after the operation, there was *no* trace of liver metastases, although the size of the tumour and lymphatic ganglion slightly increased.[76]

4. A 78-year-old male with colon cancer and liver metastases was operated on in 1978 and again in 1979. Liver mestastases were discovered in 1982, upon which biological therapy, a strict cancer diet, and Sanumgerman therapy was initiated. After one year, there were no metastases in a clinical examination, which was the same situation a further three years later.[119]

5. A 54-year-old man, with a large bean-size cancerous growth on the right lung, after taking anticancer drugs lost his appetite and was losing his strength. Five weeks after taking 500 mg daily Ge-132, X-rays showed absolutely no trace of cancer, the dry cough had disappeared, and his overall condition improved to his former state of good health.[2]

These few case histories represent a small fraction of the 'anecdotal' evidence that has accumulated, attesting to organic germanium's therapeutic effectiveness in treating cancer. Not all cancer patients receiving organic germanium have been cured; minimal therapeutic effect has been noted in several clinical trials with intravenously administered Spirogermanium. As is discussed in Chapter 13, this may in part reflect the trial selection and administration procedures.

However, almost invariably a general overall improvement in the quality of life occurs, due in large part to organic germanium's ability to relieve pain. Anecdotal case histories are not considered by scientists to be proof of a substance's efficacy, because it cannot be rigorously proved that the patient was cured by the particular substance in question. Greater agreement about methodology in clinical testing must occur if an integration between Western science and holistic medicine can occur. Holistic medicine takes the approach that the true healer is the individual himself, who, in taking whatever treatment he does, is enabling his body's own healing powers to restore him to health. Combining scientific rigour with holistic compassion will increase an individual's course of therapeutic progress.

CHAPTER 8

Germanium and arthritis

Arthritis the enigma

Recently, a programme in the BBC series 'Wider Horizons' compiled a compelling documentary of the search for the cause and ultimately a cure for one of the most debilitating diseases, rheumatoid arthritis. It included archaeological data from skeletal remains to make the point that this form of arthritis was unknown until comparatively modern times which implicates factors of our present civilization in this disease. The course of this tale took us through searches for a bacteriological and viral agent, psychological, dietary and environmental contributors, as well as malfunctioning genes, all the while poignantly demonstrating our pitiful inability to offer sustained relief for the millions of arthritis sufferers. Maniacal excitement first generated by the 'miracle cure' cortisone eventually gave way to despair, as the severe side-effects of steroids became manifest. Today, treatment for arthritis is still empirical at best, with patients having to cope, day by day, with the painful effects of this illness.

Certain forms of arthritis are the result of an 'autoimmune' disorder. The synovium, the membrane surrounding a joint, becomes inflamed, resulting in a build-up of lymphoid cells, resulting in the degeneration of bone, cartilage, ligaments, and tendons. Some agent, perhaps the Epstein–Barr virus, may trigger the initial joint inflammation, resulting in the production of antibodies. Now this is where the gene factor comes in. The product of a congenitally defective gene then alters this antibody so that it is recognized as foreign to the body. The immune system then mounts a massive defence against this factor. This immune response gone awry results in the painful swelling and inflammation characterized by arthritis. Due to the autoimmune characteristics of rheumatoid arthritis, immunosuppressive measures usually help to alleviate the pain, although sometimes with drastic effects. Interestingly, doctors have long observed that during pregnancy women's arthritis often subsides, presumably due to immunosuppressive factors that may be involved in preventing her body from 'rejecting' that of her foetus.

Metals have been used since the 1920s to treat rheumatoid arthritis. These include gold, platinum, ruthenium, and metallocene. Organic germanium has been used in animal and human clinical studies. In addition to the encouraging results emerging, there is a growing understanding of the mechanisms underlying the success of organic germanium. Thus, again, scientific progress has proceeded synchronously with holistic use, with the result that we have some insight into how germanium works.

Animal studies point out immune ——— parameters of germanium ———

The immunology group of Smith Kline & French Laboratories, directed by Michael DiMartino, has been conducting studies to evaluate the anticancer and antiarthritic properties of Spirogermanium.[21] The arthritis studies have used rats, in which arthritis is experimentally induced by a single injection of a bacterium (*Mycobacterium butyricum*) into the left hind-paw foot-pad of male rats. The primary lesion is the inflammation induced in the injected leg; the secondary lesion is the inflammation in the non-injected leg 16 days later. The results were as follows:

1. The development of both primary and secondary lesions was inhibited (17 per cent and 27 per cent respectively) by oral administration of Spirogermanium.
2. Spirogermanium administered during a 27-day period significantly suppressed hind-leg lesions on established hind-leg inflammation. Furthermore, the injected hind-leg lesions remained significantly suppressed for the 17 days following the drug treatment. The non-injected inflammation tended to increase in the post-drug period.
3. Spirogermanium restored enhanced levels of IL-1 to normal levels. IL-1, present in the synovial fluid of patients with chronic inflammation, is a product of activated macrophages involved in

immunoregulation and the stimulation of synovial cells to produce collagenase and prostaglandins.

4. Spirogermanium can induce or enhance suppressor cell activity *in vivo* in both non-arthritic as well as arthritic rats. These induced suppressor cells are radiation resistant.[4] Defective suppressor cell activity has been implicated in the pathogenesis of autoimmune diseases such as rheumatoid arthritis.

These studies suggest mechanisms to explain organic germanium's antiarthritic activity. First of all, organic germanium may work on arthritis through modulating macrophage functions, which are involved in inflammation and immunoregulation. The inhibition of macrophage functions could interfere with antigen presentation to helper T cells which could lead to the induction of suppressor cells. Also, the inhibition of IL-1 production in the inflamed joint could result in the reduction of local inflammation and tissue destruction.

Clinical trials

Seventeen patients with rheumatoid arthritis were treated with either Ge-132 alone or with small doses (under 5 mg per day) of prednisone.[1] Immune parameters were monitored, including circulating lymphocytes, T and B lymphocytes, natural killer (NK) cell activity, interferon, and antibody dependent cell mediated cytotoxicity (ADCC). The results of this study were as follows:

1. Clinical improvement of joint pains and morning stiffness were observed in 14 out of 17 patients.
2. Ge-132 treatment normalized reduced T lymphocytes, ADCC, NK cell activity, as well as interferon activity.

The conclusions reached in this study were that 'Ge-132 is useful in ...rheumatic disorders as an immunomodulator of immuno-suppressive treatment'.

CHAPTER 9

Germanium: wholeness imparted in mental illness

Each human organism represents a sum total of genetic, physical, spiritual, and environmental potential; every individual is a unique expression of life. The tremendous explosion of knowledge over the past few decades in the fields of psychology, neurochemistry, physiology, and immunology has revealed what sages have been saying for millenia, and which modern physics corroborates—that every particle of matter, every cell, every system, is intrinsically connected to every other bit of matter. The body's functioning, which includes our physical and mental state of health, is intricately influenced by thoughts of the mind, emotions, and a complex chemical transmitter network of the brain, endocrine, and immune systems. In fact, mystics and now physicists and neuro-physiologists also say that the world as we perceive it is illusory, that we are dreaming, and that all that is needed to wake up is a shift in awareness or perception. It becomes difficult to define mental illness, when so many components contribute to our actions.

The behaviours we adopt, although sometimes bizarre and self-destructive or violent, can often be understood from an archetypal psychological perspective.[6] We harbour illusions of who we are, preferring to acknowledge the 'light', the good, the strong, the nice, the unselfish. We are repelled, refuse to, or are unwilling to, admit to experience, and own the 'shadow', the bad, the vulnerable, the anger, the jealousy, all the 'nasty' elements that are also part of the human psyche. To protect ourselves from painful or traumatic experiences we may defensively fabricate an artificial shield around our darker feelings and impulses. We may become polite, good, and compliant to authority, rather than expressing our anger, resentment, or jealousy. However, for every action there is an opposite reaction, or stated another way, we harbour a memory for every thought, feeling, or action that we experience.

Sometimes these memories become locked in the body. We become 'uptight' with a stiff neck, back, and posture. Or we develop stomach ulcers from anxiety, or we have a heart attack from compulsive competitiveness and stress, or get cancer from an internal judgement of our unworthiness to be alive. The media bombards us with stories of people who suddenly go beserk and kill innocent people in a rampage. If we are truly honest with ourselves, and ask 'could I ever do such a thing?' the answer probably emerges that, under conditions of incredible stress, there is probably a trigger in all of us that could do unspeakable things. Witness the atrocities of our civilization: biblical wars, Ghengis Khan, Julius Caesar, Napoleon, Stalin, Hitler, Vietnam, etc.

Often we develop unconscious, ritualistic forms of behaviour which we cannot control—we overeat, vomit, become addicted to tobacco, alcohol, promiscuity, fear commitment and intimacy, become chronically depressed, or even develop and live in a fantasy world of our own creation.[115] These types of behaviour, which we all exhibit to greater or lesser degrees, are certainly reflections of a less than balanced mental state, but the steps necessary for restoration will probably involve changes in all aspects of our life—the food we eat, our psychological conditioning, physical care of our body, as well as any 'treatment' rendered by a health practitioner.

Mental illness is, therefore, not an isolated condition caused by a single factor. It is the manifestation of disturbances to the entire organism which can be due to many factors, such as genetic, biochemical, nutritional, psychological, etc. Therefore, approaches to these conditions must be multi-faceted, and aimed at restoring balance. However, not all 'mental' conditions require complex or esoteric techniques for dramatic improvement. In recent decades, extensive research has revealed biochemical and nutritional connections in various mental disorders, namely depression and schizophrenia.[80]

For example, excessive copper levels in the body, derived perhaps from water passing through copper pipes, copper cooking utensils, the contraceptive pill, vitamin C or B3 deficiency, can induce paranoia and hallucinations. Many depressed and schizophrenic people, severely deficient in zinc and vitamin B6, experience a multitude of symptoms including blinding headaches, nervous exhaustion, hypersensitivity to normal daylight, and nausea. Autistic children respond well to zinc and vitamin B6 therapy, and skin infections such as acne, eczema, and herpes may also improve. Cerebral allergies, a possible cause of some types of schizophrenia, respond to methionine (an amino acid), calcium, zinc, manganese, vitamins B6 and C.[80] Mood swings can be caused by allergies to common foods like wheat and to imbalances in blood sugar levels, which can be alleviated through nutritional means. It is, in all likelihood, probable that many forms of destructive and violent behaviour may have a nutritional and biochemical basis.

Organic germanium has been successfully used to treat chronic psychosis, depression, and epilepsy, and several case histories from the Asai Research Clinic are summarized below.[2]

1. A 15-year-old girl, diagnosed as being schizophrenic, became autistic, started to distrust everything, and began to be absent from school. After one month of taking organic germanium, her menstrual pains disappeared, her facial expression brightened, and her personality became cheerful. She returned to school after one year's absence.

2. A 27-year-old female suffered from depressive psychosis following an appendectomy. Her eyes appeared vacant and were full of tears. Within two days of taking 80 mg organic germanium per day, her eyes became alert. Two days later her complexion returned to normal and hardly any speech impediment remained. Ten days later she sat for her annual university examination. After 25 days, treatment was discontinued. There has been no recurrence of symptoms seven years later.

3. A 38-year-old male experienced a second seizure of depressive psychosis. His eyes appeared vacant, and he did not speak; he had been taking the drug Tofranil. He took 100 mg organic germanium twice per day. After one week, his eyes appeared brighter, although he still complained of lethargy. He reduced the Tofranil dosage to a half. Two weeks later, his eyes had returned to almost normal, and after another month he returned to work. He continued to take organic germanium for almost one year. No recurrence of symptoms has been observed for three years.

4. A 58-year-old woman had repeated periods of depressive psychosis at six monthly intervals, initially lasting for up to three months and becoming progressively worse, culminating in her

attempted suicide. Within two to three days after beginning to take 10 mg organic germanium twice per day, her persistent insomnia lifted, and the symptoms of depressive psychosis virtually vanished. She continued to take organic germanium for three years. Over the last eight years (at the time of writing), no recurrence of symptoms had been observed.

5. This 69-year-old woman had a 30-year history of depressive psychosis, seasonally coinciding with cold weather. She began to take 70 mg organic germanium twice per day. After three years of no symptoms, she discontinued organic germanium treatment. Following a cataract operation, she experienced a relapse into her former symptoms, and resumed organic germanium about five months later. She improved soon, was able to sleep through the night and experiences good health today.

The physiological and biochemical basis of how organic germanium acts to effect improvement in these various disorders has not been rigorously established. However, a careful appraisal of organic germanium's properties provides reasonable grounds to infer why this substance can be so effective for 'mental' illness.

1. First, and perhaps foremost, is organic germanium's oxygen enriching effect (see also Chapter 4). Oxygen is absolutely vital for life, and brain cells, deprived of oxygen for only three minutes, will die. The effect of increasing the brain's oxygen supply in itself is probably a great factor in organic germanium's therapeutic effects upon 'mental' disorders.

2. Organic germanium is also a powerful antioxidant (see also Chapter 4) which enables this substance to neutralize toxic free radical species, thus helping to prevent peroxidation damage to lipid membranes and having a cleansing effect on the blood quality. This overall purification effect, with the elimination of toxins, would certainly improve many so-called 'mental' disorders.

3. Organic germanium's ability to capture and discharge heavy metals (see also Chapter 5), such as mercury and cadmium which have known severe neurological effects, provides another explanation for this trace mineral's salutory effect in improving mental illnesses.

4. Another presumably major contributory factor is organic germanium's immuno-enhancing properties (see also Chapter 3). The immune system, as we have seen, is actually a complex web of organs and hormones distributed all over the body. The

enhancement of immune functions—interferon, natural killer cells, macrophages and T suppressor cells—would have a profound influence on many other biochemical and neurochemical substances, which would also be positively and naturally affected, since it is the body's own natural immune mechanisms that have been stimulated.

Because of organic germanium's therapeutic properties which seem to act at a fundamental life-enhancing level, it has been useful in treating autoimmune illnesses which also demonstrate psychiatric symptomology, such as lupus erythematosus, and possibly AIDS. Improved hormonal and immune function would certainly have a positive effect on an individual's mental health and behaviour.

Much remains to be learned about organic germanium's metabolism, biochemistry, and indeed its essentiality to the body. Detailed nutritional research into organic germanium's connection, on its own and in combination with other nutrients, with 'mental' illness could reveal even more therapeutic aspects of this trace element.

CHAPTER 10

Therapeutic ——— effects on ——— other conditions

——— Can germanium 'cure' every illness? ———

The clinical literature contains case histories in which organic germanium has been therapeutically successful in treating a wide range of illnesses and conditions. This literature spans reports from the Asai Germanium Clinic in Japan, clinical practitioners throughout Europe, and scientists and clinicians in the US.

Within the scientific and medical tradition, case histories are regarded as anecdotal evidence of a substance's efficacy, due to the lack of a controlled study, and therefore an inability to rigorously ascertain that the particular substance in question was responsible for the patient's improvement. Although rigorous, controlled studies are invaluable and perhaps indispensable in determining the therapeutic value of a substance, there is little sense in ignoring the information obtained from case studies, which can often provide the basis for more detailed research in an area.

Because of the relatively recent discovery of organic germanium as a therapeutic agent, and the major research emphasis upon its cancer-healing attributes, information for many of its other therapeutic effects is still primarily contained in laboratory research and clinic case studies, which still constitute preliminary evidence. However, at this time, controlled clinical trials are ongoing in Japan for many types of illnesses, which hopefully can more fully document organic germanium's effects on other conditions.

In view of organic germanium's action at a fundamental body level which acts to restore homeostasis by a variety of health-enhancing effects—oxygenation, immune modulation, free radical scavenging—it is not surprising that this trace element can exert such a powerful effect in so many serious conditions. This chapter highlights germanium's efficacy in treating a variety of conditions not already covered in this book.

Candida albicans

Organogermanium compounds, particularly trialkylgermanium acetates have demonstrated significant antifungal and antimicrobial activity in research studies.[94] Bacteria which were inhibited by organic germanium included *Streptococcus lactis* and *Mycobacterium phlei*.

At fairly low concentrations (100 μg/ml), organic germanium inhibited growth of a variety of fungi, including *Candida albicans*, the proliferative yeast organism which can cause thrush. Yeast infections often follow courses of antibiotic treatment, due to the disruption of the body's microbial flora balance, and systemic yeast infections often occur in AIDS patients. The application of non-toxic organic germanium as an antifungal agent would present a most promising therapeutic alternative to drugs such as nystatin, which are not always effective.

The basis of this antimicrobial and antifungal activity is most likely organic germanium's oxygenation properties. Yeast organisms thrive in low oxygen (anaerobic) environments and are killed by oxygen. Organic germanium augments metabolic oxygen levels which discourage the growth of pathogenic fungal organisms such as *Candida*.

Malaria

Malaria, a disease caused by various strains of the protozoan *Plasmodium* and transmitted by the *Anopheles* mosquito, has plagued huge areas of the world, including Africa, South America, and the Asian continent. The symptoms of malaria involve sweats, fever, and delirium, which correlate with the timing of each release of a new generation of parasites in the victim's bloodstream. The massive spraying of mosquito breeding grounds during the 1950s with DDT and other insecticides did temporarily appear to have 'eradicated' malaria. However, the development of resistant strains of the parasite to these various chemicals has resulted in the re-emergence of malaria throughout the world. Developing a vaccine has proved to be a tricky problem, due to the parasite's successful strategy of evading the body's immune system. The traditional antimalarial drug is chloroquine; however, the parasite has developed resistance to this chemical.

Mrema et al.[73] documented the antimalarial activity of Spirogermanium. The abstract from this paper is excerpted here:

> Spirogermanium... has revealed significant *in vitro* activity against chloroquine-resistant (FCB, FTA, FVO) and sensitive (FSL, FUI, FH) strains of *Plasmodium falciparum*. Inhibition of the growth and maturation of parasites after 36-h exposures to Spirogermanium started at concentrations ranging from 2.48 to 9.9 nM/ml. These concentrations appear to be within the range of Spirogermanium plasma levels reported in clinical studes with this drug. Since its clinical toxicities are unusually low in comparison with other anticancer drugs, our results on its *in vitro* activity against *Plasmodium falciparum* indicate Spirogermanium is an antimalarial drug of entirely novel structure, active in resistant strains.

The rights to Spirogermanium are owned by a New Jersey based company, Unimed, who are continuing research of Spirogermanium in several areas, including tropical medicine. There have been no other reports in the published literature about organic germanium's therapeutic effects in malaria since the above-quoted study. In view of the devastating impact, world-wide, of malaria, developing a non-toxic and effective antimalarial drug is an area certainly deserving thorough study and research.

Senile osteoporosis

Senile osteoporosis, shrinking of the total bone mass, is characterized by bone fragility and increased incidence of fracture. Bone is composed essentially of collagen, calcium and phosphate and is in a dynamic state of constant resorption and formation. Bone mass is positively correlated with blood levels of the hormones estradiol, testosterone and active cholecalciferol (previously called vitamin D_3 and inversely related to levels of parathyroid hormone (PTH)).

A 12-month study of patients with senile osteoporosis was conducted at Tokyo University, using a bone mineral analyser to determine bone mineral content.[70] Bone mass decreased in the control group of patients, while in those individuals given 1,500 mg Ge-132 daily, bone mass increased with significant differences seen one to three months from the start of taking Ge-132. The researchers considered that Ge-132 prevents bone mass decrease with ageing. Usually serum levels of PTH are high in senile osteoporosis patients;

however, Ge-132 significantly reduced serum PTH levels. Therefore the researchers postulate that organic germanium's therapeutic effect in preventing bone mass decrease is exerted by decreasing serum levels of PTH.

This study demonstrates that organic germanium exerts both a therapeutic and preventative effect upon senile osteoporosis, which can be of significant positive value for all ageing people prone to this condition.

——— Heart disease and angina pectoris ———

The following are summaries of case studies from Dr Asai's book.[2]

1. A 66-year-old man suffered from sclerotic heart disease, with chest pains, bradycardia, and slow pulse. Upon administration of Ge-132, the patient felt relief from the chest pains, and although still having difficulty walking, was able to climb a slope without frequent rests.
2. In one case of angina pectoris, where coronary dilators were not effective, organic germanium relieved the pain within a couple of days, and reduced the frequency of attacks from two or three times per day to almost nil. Attacks resumed upon stopping the administration of organic germanium.
3. One case of cardiac infarction involved a 45-year-old male suffering an attack of sharp chest pain. A large dose of organic germanium was administered; the pain subsided within a few minutes, and he fell asleep. ECGs taken over a period of three days showed 'astonishing' improvement by the third day. The man recovered and was able to work normally.

—— Circulatory problems—Raynaud's Disease ——

Raynaud's disease is a disease of the circulation, in which gangrene develops in the limbs, sometimes requiring amputation. Several successful cases treated with Ge-132 are reported from Dr Asai's clinic, describing how, following the administration of organic germanium, gangrene was markedly reduced, and rosy colour restored, denoting good blood circulation.[2]

——————————— Eye diseases ———————————

Organic germanium has been successfully used to treat eye diseases including glaucoma, black cataracts, detached retinas, and inflammation of the retina and optic nerves. It is stated in Dr Asai's book that 'germanium rejuvenates retinal vessels, and is therefore effective in treating glaucoma and amaurosis (partial or total blindness).'[2] This area certainly is a fertile one for rigorous study.

Epilepsy

There are reports both of Ge-132 and Sanumgerman having success with epilepsy in children. In a report of a 16-year-old boy taking Sanumgerman, there was an initial dramatic improvement in which for ten days there were no fits. Then, after a fortnight, a fit occurred, and gradually they became as frequent as before the treatment. Increase in the dosage resulted in some improvement but the initial success was never reattained.[42]

Due to the difficulties involved with epilepsy, and the severely toxic effects of most of the available medication, this certainly points to yet another area to investigate more closely.

The common cold?

Organic germanium's anti-viral and immuno-enhancing properties enable speculation as to its possible preventative and therapeutic effects upon the common cold. This is certainly an area open to clinical research.

Other diseases

Conditions which have responded to treatment with organic germanium include chronic gastritis, influenza, Parkinson's disease, cerebral sclerosis, burns and multiple sclerosis.

CHAPTER 11

Safety of organic ——— germanium ——— products

The exemplary record
——— of organic germanium's safety ———

There is a long and drawn-out process of testing required in order that a substance can be marketed as a drug. This involves efficacy tests in animals, elaborate toxicity studies in animals, teratogenic studies in animals, testing on human volunteers, then a tier of clinical trials in humans. These requirements, in addition to providing the public with some assurance of safety, also contribute to the long lead time and enormous expense of new product development.

All the organic germanium compounds discussed here—Sanumgerman, Ge-132 and Spirogermanium—have been subjected to rigorous testing, including all the above steps, and have been found to be virtually non-toxic, except that Spirogermanium has been found to cause transient nervous side-effects. At present, Spirogermanium is being developed for use as a drug, while Sanumgerman and Ge-132 are available as nutritional supplements. This may change in the future; it is possible that organic germanium may become classified as a prescription drug at higher doses.

Organic germanium is also somewhat unusual, although by no means unique, in that its creator, Dr Asai, tested the initially synthesized product on himself, cured his arthritis, and distributed it to others who also were therapeutically helped. Then extensive testing was carried out, which confirmed the empirical and insightful determinations that this substance was non-toxic. That organic germanium is a naturally occurring substance and could be regarded as a food supplement, made this approach feasible and probably accelerated the research and clinical findings many-fold. If organic germanium had been initially viewed as a new drug, it probably would have had to undergo years of animal tests before being given to humans for testing.

What happens to
—— organic germanium in the body ——

Organic germanium compounds are rapidly absorbed and eliminated from the body without undergoing metabolic alteration. Studies have been performed which trace the route that organic germanium follows in its 'trip' through the body.[58,70] The studies performed with the various compounds have yielded essentially similar data with respect to absorption, distribution, and elimination rates from the body, and the following incorporates the data from all the compounds.

Within one hour of administration, 50 per cent of the compound is in the gastrointestinal tract; after twelve hours, only 5 per cent is there. Organic germanium is resorbed by the vena portae. One hour after administration, 50 per cent is in the vena portae; after eight hours, this figure rises to 85 per cent and by twelve hours, it is quasi-complexed. Serum plasma levels reach a maximum two hours after administration, in eight hours, germanium is reduced by 80 per cent of the maximum.

Organic germanium, administered orally, has also been shown to be absorbed by about 30 per cent distributed evenly throughout the body, leaving almost no residual concentration after 12 hours. It is excreted, unchanged metabolically, in the urine in 24 hours. Germanium is ubiquitously distributed in all organs—there are no specific target organs, and no differences in distribution patterns detected between sexes.

Organic germanium is also eliminated at quite a rapid, linear rate, of approximately 8 per cent of the dose per hour, during the first eight hours. It is completely eliminated after three days, mainly via the kidneys (85 per cent). Germanium is soluble in the interstitial fluids, and is not protein bound. Germanium does not accumulate in any organ (see, however, below)—no germanium can be found in animals one week after their removal from treatment.

—— Animal toxicity studies ——

Animal toxicity studies measure doses and effecs of a substance administered and determine levels at which damage, or indeed death, occurs. Sanumgerman and Ge-132 were both found to be totally non-toxic when administered orally, up to 3.4 g/kg and 10 g/kg respectively in mice and rats.[2,85] This is a huge amount of organic germanium, which was not found to cause any detectable abnormal effects.

Chronic toxicity studies were carried out in rats for six months with both Ge-132 and Sanumgerman,[2,85] with the animals receiving varying doses of the respective organic germanium compound. At the termination of the study, an extensive range of parameters was measured, to assess whether the administration of organic germanium over a protracted period caused any abnormalities. These parameters included general condition, appearance, behaviour, motor activity, appetites, body weight, biochemical assays of blood serum, haemoglobin, red cells, leukocytes, platelets, weight of internal organs, macroscopic and microscopic appearance of internal organs, respiration, blood pressure, intestinal tonus, and contractility. In totally independent studies, performed in different parts of the world, with both these organic germanium compounds, no abnormalities in any of these parameters were found.

——————— Human toxicity studies ———————

In human clinical trials with healthy volunteers, as well as patients who have participated in all the studies described throughout this book, the toxicity of the particular organic germanium compound was assessed.[69] One of the outstanding features of organic germanium is its virtual non-toxicity and its ability to be tolerated, in contrast to most highly toxic drugs. Even Spirogermanium, which seemed to generate mainly neurological symptoms, was remarked to be well tolerated. However, it is difficult to directly compare Spirogermanium to Ge-132 and Sanumgerman, because it has mainly been administered intravenously in human patients.

In the large number of cases histories and clinical trials reported, there are very few reports of any symptomology developing as a result of oral organic germanium administration. Taken orally, organic germanium is highly safe.

——— Mutagenic and teratogenic studies ———

Mutagenicity studies assess a compound's ability to cause mutations to the DNA of an organism. In controlled studies by the method of Ames, Sanumgerman was found NOT to be a mutagenic agent.[30] Teratogenic studies assess any damage to developing foetuses caused by administration of a substance to pregnant mothers. Ge-132 has been assessed for teratogenicity in mice, rats and rabbits;

Sanumgerman (an older formulation) in rats. For both these organic germanium compounds, there were no noted abnormalities in the pregnant females. With some doses of both these compounds, there were some differences in the weight of foetuses and the ratio of absorbed foetuses, and skeletal abnormalities were observed.[2,22] Skeletal malformations also occurred in the control group.

It is difficult to accurately extrapolate between animals and humans. In teratogenic studies, animals are often given rather high doses of a substance, higher than a human would probably ingest. However, despite Dr Asai's assertions of the benefits of taking organic germanium during pregnancy, the demonstration of even slight teratogenic activity in animals should be borne in mind when considering taking any substance during pregnancy.

Toxicity of contaminated
——— organic germanium compounds ———

There is a single report in the literature of a women who had been taking germanium compound over a protracted period and who died of renal failure.[74] This woman had been taking 600 mg per day of a germanium compound for over 18 months as an elixir. Following her death, analysis of the compound revealed mainly germanium dioxide (GeO_2), with some organic germanium compound. An autopsy revealed gross cellular abnormalities of kidney tissues and an increased accumulation of germanium in several organs. It was not possible to determine whether the germanium compound had caused renal failure, or whether renal failure had caused the accumulation of the germanium, since Ge is eliminated mainly by the kidneys.

Study of the older toxicity literature, spanning the 1920s to the 1950s, which investigated the toxicity of mainly inorganic germanium[41,83,89,90,113], reveals that, properly buffered and administered in sublethal doses, inorganic germanium is not always damaging; however, in some cases, shock and death occurred to animals administered inorganic germanium. The Japanese woman, mentioned above, had been taking a compound composed mainly of inorganic germanium, and had suddenly taken ill and died. Although this is the only reported case ever of the accumulation of germanium, it should not be dismissed necessarily as coincidence; it should be borne in mind that inorganic forms of germanium may be toxic in high doses.

─── Organic germanium is safe ───

The rigorous tests described above demonstrate the safety of taking even very large doses of organic germanium. Doses of more than 10 g/kg body weight produced no damaging effects in rats. A very large therapeutic dose, administered for cancer patients may be 1 g per day, obviously much less than that given to the rats.

Many of the most common substances we ingest, including aspirin, and even some supplements such as selenium, have toxic properties. It is said that if many of our older medications were forced to undergo the rigours of present-day testing, they would fail. In the light of this, apart from the suggested caution during pregnancy, organic germanium, even taken at high dosages, is certainly safe.

CHAPTER 12

Issues of interest to —— the consumer of —— organic germanium

Why hasn't germanium —— been heard of before now? ——

Many individuals outside the nutritional and clinical research fields may never have heard of germanium before, except perhaps as the material that transistors used to be made of. I had not heard of the therapeutic effects of this trace element until I began to delve into the literature that has accumulated over the last decade. I have been puzzled by the fact that information about this substance has not been more generally available before the present time. A combination of factors, including the following, are probably responsible:

1. Researchers in the various clinics, companies and laboratories have been preoccupied in their research, developing their product or testing the substance. Much of this research has been performed in Japan, where organic germanium has been more widely available and familiar to the public. Their research results were, however, published in the scientific literature, which is in the public domain.

2. Individuals doing corporate research, for propriety purposes, maintain a fairly high degree of confidentiality in their research.

3. There is usually a lag time before information in the scientific journals gets 'translated' into the more general literature. It is simply a matter of time before a certain 'critical mass' of

information accumulates to enable people to put together the various pieces of individual research.

The 'pieces' of the germanium puzzle started to come together at the First International Conference on Germanium, organized by Sanum—Kehlbeck and held at Hanover, West Germany in October 1984. This brought together researchers from Japan, Europe, and the US to discuss the various aspects of organic germanium. Since then the Germanium Research Department of the International Institute of Symbiotic Studies has been created in the UK, and North American nutritionists have formed the Germanium Institute of North America (GINA) to disseminate information and further clinical research with organic germanium.[47,49]

This international co-operation of scientists, clinicians, and nutritionists in the field of organic germanium research has had a synergistic effect in furthering clinical research and disseminating information to the public about the health-enhancing effects of this substance.[31–33,45,48,66]

—————— Germanium content in food ——————

In 1967, Shroeder and Balassa published a paper[91] which documented that germanium is biologically ubiquitous. They surveyed all manner of biological material, from seafood (oysters, clams, shrimp, salmon, tuna, etc.), meat (pork, chicken, beef, lamb), dairy products, grains (rye, wheat, rice, oats), vegetables (beans, carrots, broccoli, cauliflower, tomato, etc.) nuts, beverages (tea, coffee, cocoa), oils, even cat food and cigarettes (Turkish and Canadian!) The data showed that germanium was present in trace amounts in most foods. Only clams, canned tuna, baked beans (the highest content with 4.67 ppm) and Welch's tomato juice contained more than 2 ppm. Daily germanium intake varied according to diet, with ovo-vegetarian and high protein diets containing 3.2 and 0.866 mg respectively.

Later analyses, using more sophisticated technology, revealed merely trace amounts of germanium in plants used for Chinese medicine.[68] This paper by Mino *et al.* has a vital bearing on all of the germanium work. These researchers used flameless atomic absorption spectrometry (AAS) combined with solvent extraction, which is a much more sensitive technique than used by either Asai or Schroeder. Some of the same medicinal plants were assayed by this procedure.

Germanium contents in medicinal plants, e.g. Ginseng radix,

selected on the basis of Asai's report, were less than 6 ppb in every case. The results obtained indicate that medicinal plants in general contain small amounts of germanium, and suggest that there may be no connection between the pharmacological effects of the medicinal plants and their germanium content... The analytical values in this experiment were much lower than those of Asai's report and even than those given in Schroeder's report. The method used by Asai was not clear. The measurements of Schroeder were... with phenylfluorone as a color-forming agent. This colorimetry (detection limit, 0.5 ppm) has such low sensitivity that the values obtained 0.1–1.0 ppm must be considered as unreliable. Therefore the germanium contents in other biomaterials should also be reinvestigated by the present procedure using flameless AAS.

Reports of high germanium content in certain plants and herbs, including garlic and ginseng, have started to appear in publications.[45] The original results obtained by Asai have been superceded by more sensitive methods, and attention should be paid so as not to perpetuate erroneous figures in the literature. The suggestion to re-evaluate the germanium content in biomaterials should be heeded, in the light of the above-quoted report. In any case, even the values obtained by Asai do not constitute therapeutic doses, which he himself acknowledged.[2]

─────── **Is germanium an essential mineral?** ───────

The average daily human intake of germanium, in the mg range, is not a minute quantity. However, germanium's essentiality as a mineral to the body's metabolism has yet to be established; thus, it cannot be ascertained what, if any, disorders may arise from a germanium deficiency. Also, there is considerable ignorance about germanium's metabolic role in the body.[110]

It was not so long ago that we were ignorant of the essential role of vitamins, minerals and trace minerals, DNA—the substance genes are made of—how genetic information is translated into proteins, the existence of elementary particles such as quarks, gluons, mesons, etc. Recognition of ignorance is often a vital first step to the establishment of any intelligent plan to find out the answer to a question.

Research, such as that reported here about the modulation by organic germanium of the glutathione enzyme complex, is a tangible step towards answering this question, as would be research assessing pathologies resulting from germanium deficiencies as well as the basic metabolism of germanium by humans and animals.

An entire area open to research investigation is the potential therapeutic effects of organic germanium on livestock. Supplementation of livestock feed with trace elements such as selenium have achieved significant effects in alleviating many serious disorders. Investigations of abundance of germanium in soils would provide much useful information that would cross-fertilize the human clinical research information.

Natural sources of germanium

As stated above, germanium is a ubiquitous trace element, and is present in almost all foodstuffs in micro-trace amounts in the ppm or ppb range. However, in order to obtain enough germanium to exert a therapeutic effect, one would have to consume enormous quantities of foods. It is this realization which drove Dr Asai to labour for almost two decades to develop a synthetic form of organic germanium, in which task he succeeded in 1967. Therefore, in order to obtain organic germanium in supplemental or therapeutic dosages, it is necessary to use organic germanium supplements.

—————————Food supplement or drug —————————

Organic germanium is virtually non-toxic and is presently being sold as a food supplement in Europe, the UK, and the US. Organic germanium's therapeutic properties might lead it to be classified as a drug in the future, depending on the complex factors and regulations governing nutritional supplements, therapeutic claims, and profits which stand to be made by organic germanium manufacturers. Were this to happen, organic germanium could be marketed more lucratively as a drug, and not be confined to the less profitable supplement market. It would definitely benefit manufacturers of organic germanium; however, consumers would no longer be able to purchase, over-the-counter, this safe and therapeutically beneficial trace mineral.

With more information being disseminated about the uses of organic germanium, consumer and practitioner pressure could probably stop organic germanium from being designated purely as a drug. This would not, of course, prevent practitioners from prescribing organic germanium to patients on prescription.

————— Patent and trademark issues —————

The Asai organization does not make any Ge-132 available for export. Therefore, any Ge-132 used outside of the Asai Germanium Clinic is manufactured from other sources. There are three patented processes for the manufacture of Ge-132 in Japan, all of which have expired in Japan. However, there is still an extant American patent for the manufacture of Ge-132, which is also the trade-marked name for the Asai form of germanium sesquioxide. The two sources of organic germanium in the UK are Global Marketing and Inpa AG. The trade names *Ge Oxy-132* and *Germanooxyd* are both registered trade-marks. Sanumgerman and similarly formulated compounds are patented internationally.

—— Why is organic germanium so expensive? ——

A first reaction to buying organic germanium could be shock at the price. The prices range from below 30p per capsule for lower dosages to well in excess of £1 per capsule for higher doses. The broadness of this price range is based on the difficulties of comparing different products containing varying amounts of elemental germanium. However, although organic germanium is still considerably more expensive than most vitamins and minerals, it is less expensive than most prescription drugs.

Germanium is expensive to extract from the earth. It is extracted as germanium concentrates from the smelting of sulphidic ores such as copper, lead and zinc, which enriches its concentration from 10 ppm to 50 ppm. Following steps such as alkaline refinement, it is enriched to 500 ppm. Several additional processes are required to obtain the raw materials for the synthesis of organic germanium. This establishes a high base price. Then it must be synthesized to the organic form, which involves complex and expensive machinery and a large number of synthesis stages. Final purification procedures necessary to bring the product up to the utmost high-grade quality are also costly. For Ge-132, if the elemental content is merely 40 per cent instead of 42 per cent, the price is reduced by one-third, but there is significant contamination by other metals. Superimposed upon this are the substantial research expenses which have been incurred to carry out tests for toxicity and therapeutic activity. At present, all the organic germanium products available are quite expensive, compared to most other supplements. In view of this product's therapeutic effects, however, it is certainly worth the price, providing that the quality is beyond reproach.

Quality of organic
—————— germanium supplements ——————

This is a most important consideration. The two types of high quality organic germanium available are the Ge-132 variety, and Sanumgerman. Inorganic germanium, such as germanium dioxide, may be toxic. Testing for purity of organic germanium samples is costly and complex. The following techniques are used:

1. NMR (Proton Nuclear Magnetic Resonance) spectroscopy.
2. IR (infra-red) spectroscopy. A combination of these two techniques provides a 'molecular fingerprint' of the molecule.
3. Elemental analysis of single elements.
4. Germanium content by AAS (Atomic Absorption Spectroscopy); X-Ray diffraction and X-Ray dispersive analyses.
5. Trace analysis to determine metallic contamination by AAS and ICP (Inductive Coupled Plasma Emission).
6. Wet chemical analyses.
7. Titration, only applied for Ge-132, assesses the amount of acid carboxyl groups present in the sample molecule, which can be compared with a fixed theoretical value.

In addition to the above, the following extra tests are performed with Sanumgerman:

1. Optical rotation of the compound in solution.
2. Enzymatic determination of citrate and lactate content.

Testing by an independent analytical laboratory of several organic germanium products available on the North American market revealed significant discrepancies between the stated elemental germanium content and what was actually found in the analysis (results disclosed to author). The deviations ranged from 25 per cent less than to 19.6 per cent more than the amount of Ge-132 which ought to have been present. Theoretically, these discrepancies could be explained by the following:

1. The capsules were not filled with the stated quantity of Ge-132.
2. The used Ge-132 compound did not contain the prescribed 42.8 per cent elemental Ge; the two extremes disclosed by the tests were 32 per cent and 51.2 per cent.

The precise methodologies necessary for accurate testing of the purity of organic germanium samples should be a matter for the industry experts to establish, standardize and maintain, in order to bring into existence international co-operation in this vital area of quality control. It behoves all the manufacturers, distributors and clinicians to establish and agree upon an international standard of testing and quality assurance for organic germanium samples.

Centres of organic
———— germanium research ————

Japan

In 1978, a nation-wide organization, composed of many research and medical institutions, was inaugurated in Japan to 'deepen the research on Ge-132 from both the fundamental and clinical aspects' (Mizushima).[70] The Japanese are currently conducting three double-blind randomized clinical trials on organic germanium's efficacy in lung and gastro-intestinal cancers, and shingles, a herpes virus disease. There have also been discussions of research with organic germanium on AIDS in Japan.

The Asai Germanium Clinic is located at Murata Building 5F, 6–4–14 Seijo Setagaya-ku, Tokyo 157.

Europe

Clinics, universities, and research centres throughout Eastern and Western Europe have been researching and clinically testing Sanumgerman for about ten years in collaboration with Sanum-Kehlbeck, Postfach 332, 2812 Hoya, West Germany. The distribution company for Sanum-Kehlbeck's organic germanium products is called Inpa AG; sole agents in the UK for Sanumgerman and Ge-132 being Symbiogenesis Ltd., BCM Box 22, London WC1 3XX.

Dr Gunter Paetz, general practitioner and homoeopath is familiar with the organic germanium research in Europe.[76] He is contactable through Sanum-Kehlbeck.

Dr Eugen Zoubek, Pares del Peru, 138A Elvira Los Lumbres, Marbella, Malaga, Spain, medical and homoeopathic doctor, is currently publishing a book documenting his extensive experience using Sanumgerman with ninety-five cancer patients, showing greater than a 70 per cent success rate.

UK

The Germanium Research Department of the International Institute of Symbiotic Studies (Monica Bryant, Director, 5 Fairlight Place, Brighton, Sussex, BN2 3AH, England) is providing a focus for the compilation and dissemination of information, quality control, education and research into the use of organic germanium for various diseases, including AIDS.[33]

Jan de Vries, naturopath at Southwood Road, Troon, Ayrshire, Scotland, met with Dr Asai in 1975 and has been using organic germanium therapeutically in his practice.

North America

Several oncology groups and the immunology group from Smith Klein & French have performed clinical trials for the organic germanium compound Spirogermanium. The rights to Spirogermanium are held by Unimed Inc., Lucien Joubert, Medical Director, 35 Columbia Road, Somerville NJ.

The Germanium Institute of North America (GINA), Parris Kidd, Director, P.O. Box 8207, Berkely, California, has a distinguished advisory board composed of individuals representing a broad range of research, clinical, orthodox and alternative medical expertise.[47]

Dr Stephen Levine, nutritionist and allergy specialist, Director, Allergy Research Group, PO Box 489, San Leandro, California, has clinical experience with organic germanium.[62, 63]

———— Advice to the consumer ————

The consumer should be well aware of the commerical competition that exists with organic germanium products, so that he/she can avoid any inferior products and demand certification of the highest quality of any organic germanium they wish to purchase.

When purchasing organic germanium, be certain that it is in fact organic and not inorganic germanium. Be especially mindful that it is of the highest quality. Ask to see the analytical specifications attesting to its purity. Deal only with reputable and honest dealers.

CHAPTER 13

Regimes for —— taking organic —— germanium

——The Asai Germanium Clinic regime——

Dr Asai believed that there are three vital elements which greatly facilitate healing: (a) the individual must be firmly convinced that he/she will get better; (b) strict attention must be paid to diet to maintain a proper acid/alkali balance; (c) great attention, including positive measures of stress reduction, should be devoted to the promotion of a healthy oxygen supply, crucial to healthy cell metabolism.

Well-balanced diet

According to the oriental dietary system, which classifies foods according to their acid or alkali-forming qualities, a healing diet is one which maintains the pH of the bodily fluids slightly alkaline at pH 7.2 to 7.4.

For those acquainted with other types of dietary regimes which may advocate seemingly contradictory advice, it is advisable not to mix different healing systems. Each healing tradition works within its own frame of reference, and as long as one is faithful to that particular frame of reference positive results are likely to be obtained. The oriental classification of foods according to their acidity or alkalinity is difficult to rationalize with Western biochemical notions of nutrition. This is a classic example of the dichotomy separating holistic and reductionist world views. Regardless of one's adherence or otherwise to this system, oriental healing diets, such as macrobiotics, have been some of the most effective against even 'terminal' illnesses such as cancer and, more recently, AIDS.

Acid-forming foods tend to acidify the blood, while alkaline foods do the reverse. In order to maintain a slightly alkaline pH, highly acidic foods should be avoided, as should excessive intake of animal fats and proteins. In general, one's diet should be centred around whole natural vegetable foods, such as grains, vegetables, fruits, etc., with an emphasis upon balance. The following table is extracted from *The Book of Whole Meals* by Annemarie Colbin.[14]

Acid forming foods	Alkalizing foods
Sugar/honey	Fruit
Oil	Potatoes
Nuts	Raw vegetables
White flour	Cooked vegetables
Fish	Sea vegetables
Fowl	Kuzu
Eggs	Fresh beans
Meat	Sea salt
Milk	Regular salt
Butter	Shoyu
Cheese	Miso

Oxygen supply/stress reduction

As discussed in Chapter 4, oxygen is not a substance to be taken for granted. An oxygen deficiency can have far-reaching toxic consequences; healing is inestimably facilitated by oxygen-promoting practices. At the Asai Germanium Clinic, an attempt is made to bring into balance the entire lifestyle of the individual, so as to maximize the natural healing abilities of the individual, which are also enhanced by organic germanium.

Stress, anxiety, fear, all can promote oxygen deficiency within the body. Practices which induce relaxation can create a glow, a harmony, an expansiveness of positive hope, a sense of fulfilment and contentment, which greatly enhances healing. Therefore, practices such as yoga, meditation, walking, breath awareness, in fact anything which is relaxing, would absolutely support any therapeutic programme.

Organic germanium

The dosages prescribed by the physicians at the Asai Germanium Clinic vary according to each individual. For serious illnesses such as cancer, high doses of organic germanium, in the range of between 500 mg and 1 gm daily are often prescribed. This may be in combinations of liquid and/or powder forms.

The Asai Germanium Clinic does not export organic germanium. In order to receive Ge-132 treatment at the Asai Clinic, it is necessary to visit there in person. The following is taken from a letter sent from the Asai Clinic regarding Ge-132 treatment:

> The doctor in charge will diagnose the present condition of the patient and examine, in detail, any previous illnesses, complications and associated conditions. The patient's age, height, weight and nourishment, ingestion, urination, defecation and sleep conditions, etc. are also checked. And if necessary, the samples of patient's urine and blood are taken for serological haematological analyses and other examinations. According to the results obtained, the daily dosage and number of doses of Ge-132 considered to be most effective for each patient are determined.
>
> In this way, Ge-132 is to be administered to the patients themselves with medical instructions necessary for the course of treatment. If the patient is not examined in detail, and daily dosage and number of doses cannot be determined and effective treatment cannot be expected. One hundred patients afflicted with the same disease have to be given completely different dosage of Ge-132 per day according to the conditions mentioned above.

European clinical regimes

Each practitioner is different and may emphasize different treatment practices. However, in examining case histories from practitioners in several European countries, several common features emerge in the course of germanium treatment of the patient.

The European practitioners prescribing organic germanium have also been practising a variety of alternative medical therapies, including oxygen/ozone therapy, vitamin, mineral, and natural therapies, dietary therapies, acupuncture and homoeopathy. Patients encompass a broad spectrum, ranging from cancer patients diagnosed as 'terminal', already having had one or more operations, and perhaps other anticancer treatments, to aged victims afflicted with arthritis and other debilitating diseases.

In the majority of case history reports which I viewed, the practitioner has usually added organic germanium to the regime of other therapies prescribed, therefore making it difficult to compare dosages of germanium prescribed, and indeed, to attribute any observed therapeutic effects solely to organic germanium. However, the practitioners with extensive experience with organic germanium have prescribed doses ranging from 200 to 1,200 mg daily, depending on the individual. Because of the variety of treatments employed, it has therefore been difficult to assess rigorously the effects of organic germanium in many instances.

US clinical trials
with Spirogermanium

Several oncology groups in North America have performed phase I and II clinical trials with Spirogermanium on patients suffering from a variety of cancers. While the *in vitro*, animal studies and phase I data with Spirogermanium are comparable to those of Ge-132 and Sanumgerman, it is interesting to note that in many of the trials, Spirogermanium frequently had limited effects on the course of the cancers.[8,11,12,19,20,24–26,46,56,81,93,106,108]

While it could be reasonably argued that these clinical trials were actually more scientific and rigorous than the clinical experience from Japan, and that they represent 'real' and 'unbiased' clinical situations, there are several factors worth noting in relation to overall clinical trial management practice employed in Western medicine in general, and with the Spirogermanium trials in particular, which may contribute to the seemingly 'inactive' results of this drug.

Patient eligibility criteria

Many patients participating in the Spirogermanium trials had been 'heavily pretreated'. This means that these individuals had already received other forms of treatment for their cancers, including possibly surgery, chemotherapy, and radiation therapy regimes, and that they had failed to respond to these other treatments. In view of the highly cytotoxic effects of some of these regimes, and the frequently devastating effects of chemotherapy and radiation treatment upon the immune system, it is hardly surprising that the Spirogermanium treatment failed to elicit a positive response.

The Spirogermanium was administered to the hospitalized individuals intravenously. This is in stark contrast to the Japanese regime where the individual is responsible for and takes an active role in his germanium treatment. The Western clinical trial procedure places a patient in a passive, virtually non-participatory role, receiving yet another treatment for his/her cancer. For an individual's belief that he will get better to play a role in the healing process, studies must be designed to enable the person to marshall the powerful healing forces of his mind. Western clinical trials whereby individuals are admitted on the basis that every other treatment has failed, hardly provide a basis for positive hope for that particular treatment.

The entire treatment model in the West makes the individual a passive spectator to the treatment of his own illness. In such cases, the objectives of scientific enquiry may be satisfied, but at the cost of the patient dying. The ultimate objective of any treatment or study must be the life and health of the individual, not the establishment of the efficacy of a particular treatment. It may be necessary to sacrifice some 'objectivity' in order to save lives; since when is this out of step with the most sacred vows of the Hippocratic oath?

CHAPTER 14

Esoteric and speculative aspects of organic germanium

Transcending the mind—entering spiritual realms

The esoteric traditions of East and West tell us that we, as conscious entities, are more than the mind. In fact, one of the fundamental illusions that has been stamped upon our brains is that the physical is all that is real. So-called transcendental or altered states of consciousness connect us with other dimensions available to us, that we can relate to with senses other than simply the logical mind. These types of experiences are not as rare or weird as often thought—most of us have felt uncommonly moved by the awe of a violent storm, the silence of a beautiful sunset, the might of a roaring river, exhilaration of speed in skiing or running, those times when so totally relaxed that we just seem to 'melt' and time stands still. These 'peak experiences' are common to all. What we may not have realized is that this experience of reality is probably more 'true' than our usual fear-dominated everyday mode of trials and tribulations which keeps us on an endless wheel of mental gymnastics and regurgitation.

The upsurge in interest in phenomena which are not easily understandable by ordinary logic has led to the active participation by many in meditation and spiritual practices which attune and access qualities which have been named psychic, intuitive, feminine—those parts of our being which can foretell disaster many miles away, which can 'feel' the breeze, marvel at the sunset, and intuit what is 'going on' in another person. To develop and pay attention to the intuitive, the spiritual, is not to refute science or logic. Rather, all of these aspects of consciousness represent the sum total of our developed awareness.

When physicists in this century were confronted with a paradigm which didn't conform to currently respected dogma, they literally had to declare ignorance—what had appeared to be, simply could not be so, according to the rules of physics. This had led physicists to adopt a position more similar, in the past, to that of the philosophers or mystics: that much of the way we view reality is an illusion. Much of western science is based upon the premise of an objective observer; this premise has been shown to be untrue. There is no such thing as an isolated, objective observer. Every particle, action, person, thing, is interconnected to the rest of the universe. This has led to the development of what has been called the holistic paradigm, a way of looking at things in their entirety, remembering that the whole is not simply the sum of all the separate parts.

Men of vision who have spanned the worlds of vision and science have always been with us and we benefit from the legacy of their ability to 'see' beyond the obvious, to 'imagine' things that simply could not be explained. In their time, Copernicus and Galileo were riduculed for postulating that the Earth was not the centre of the universe. Leonardo da Vinci had the vision to design a flying machine centuries before this marvel became a reality. Kekule literally 'dreamed' the vision from whence came the resonance theory in chemistry. Even the discovery of penicillin can be partly attributed to the farsightedness of Alexander Fleming not throwing away the fuzzy petri dish with the white mould growing on it. Almost all the great discoveries were probably thought impossible at the time they were proposed. This simply reflects the limited capacity of our left-brain to go beyond what is known into the unknown. Science at its essence is a great leap into and exploration of the unknown. True expansive science, which utilizes all our faculties, is at one with magic, alchemy, the historical pursuit of great art and creation.

The healing abilities of —— organic germanium defy normal logic ——

Organic germanium appears to be able to effect therapeutic benefit in almost every illness imaginable. This in itself makes this substance highly suspect to our sceptical mind, it almost seems too good to be true, and therefore could be considered to be yet another phoney 'miracle' cure. However, in this case, the rigorous scientific evidence to date of its efficacy pinpoints properties which are proven and understandable scientifically. Therefore we have measured and can verify organic germanium's immuno-enhancing, oxygen-enriching, free radical scavenging, and analgesic properties. Good. But, what if we go beyond the purely logical, measurable entities and entertain speculation about other non-physical properties of this element germanium which may also help to explain some of its 'elixir'-like qualities? It is not necessary to believe in esoterica to entertain speculation—merely to suspend disbelief. The truth is that we don't really know all there is to know about germanium; perhaps in speculating we will come closer to the truth and discover more of its secrets.

——— Is organic germanium an elixir? ———

Dr Asai had the original insight and conceived the idea of organic germanium being of therapeutic value in the body, and also worked for decades as a researcher to actually synthesize the organic form of this element. Dr Asai says about this substance:

> My connection with germanium started by chance, certainly, but I cannot help perceiving there a working of some supernormal inevitability...when I review the seventy-odd years of my life, I seem to find a consistent thread or a command from some outside source that transcends my own will which has determined my continued research of this amazing compound...it is a substance understandable only through high level meditative deliberations with a highly sharpened mind...when I gaze upon the single crystal of germanium with its silver-grey sheen, I have the illusion of seeing my whole life crystallized in this substance; I also feel, on the palm of my hand, the touch of a substance I am tempted to describe as the fountain of life that fills the universe.[2]

The notion of an elixir is as old as man himself. It is the much sought-after quest for the philosopher's stone, of transmuting base metals into gold, of the substance which if drunk, could grant eternal youth and life. Is there substance to this quest, or are these mere fairy tales? The alchemical formulae for the philospher's stone are well-guarded secrets granted only to those initiates entitled to the knowledge; however, certain principles have come down to us through the ages which offer a useful point of departure when attempting to discuss organic germanium as a potential elixir.

One criterion for the elixir substance is that it be from the earth, an ore, a metal. Germanium certainly fulfils this property. Also, that during its transmutation it be 'fired' to be purified. Germanium is extracted during the smelting of zinc and copper ores. Continuing on in this vein, that during an intermediate stage it be a white crystalline substance, soluble in water. Organic germanium is a white crystalline substance, water soluble. Not being an accomplished alchemist, I cannot talk with great authority of organic germanium being an elixir; however, I point out these qualities which bear a striking resemblance to the age-old alchemical mysteries and thus perhaps inspire contemplation of this element's ultimate potential.

Germanium is a crystal

Crystals embody energies which can be effectively channelled for insight and healing. The healing properties of crystals are becoming well known, and many people are learning to attune and utilize these healing energies for personal and planetary healing. The healing nature of crystals is thought to be derived from 'energy' fields, which ultimately are a consequence of electrons creating these energy fields.[7] Organic germanium in its solid form is a crystal, and, of course, one of the most fundamental properties of germanium is its semiconductor nature, its ability to donate and receive electrons easily. Many of organic germanium's healing properties may be due to its intrinsic electronic qualities.

Germanium and energy fields

When attempting to rationalize how a substance can actually work to alleviate the symptoms of many diverse illnesses, I have over and over again returned to the concept of somehow altering the electric potential, the energy field of an individual. In Chinese medicine, chi or ki is the energy field. When an individual is sick, his energy is 'blocked', and treatments such as acupuncture can 'unblock' and bring his energy into alignment, or balance, where healing can occur.

Could it be that organic germanium is actually working at a fundamental energy level of the body, helping to restore balance to a system out of balance?

Recently some experimental results were communicated to me by an electro-acupuncturist from Germany, who has been using a methodology according to Dr Reinhold Voll, which has intricately calibrated settings on the electrical scale with corresponding conditions. In these reported electro-acupuncture experiments, various foods, flour, grain, and bread caused severe pain and allergic reaction. When the grain and flour were soaked in germanium water, the points were no longer painful and appeared to reach equilibrium.

If, in addition to being soaked in germanium water, the bread, grain, flour, and water were also placed in a magnetic field of 40 hertz, the substances not only were not painful, but also insecticides could no longer be detected.

Other experiments documenting organic germanium's biophysical properties have been performed,[54] pointing to this substance's ability to influence energetic and magnetic properties.

It is intriguing, albeit still premature, to link germanium's action with those of energetic healing phenomena which work with the 'subtle energy fields' of the body.

CHAPTER 15

A practical
——— guide to ———
holistic living

Organic germanium—enhancing our health
——————— and our lives ———————
This book has attempted to bring together the many aspects currently known regarding the therapeutic uses of organic germanium. The topics covered span a wide range of issues and illnesses, including environmental pollution from radiation and heavy metals, modulation of the immune and nervous system, and some of the presently not understood and esoteric properties of organic germanium, which suggest that its healing abilities may work at levels beyond the physical.

Organic germanium as a substance seems to enhance and enrich our health, and restore balance to whatever system is 'diseased'. Really, in a nutshell, this is what holistic living is all about—learning and knowing about ourselves and our fellow earthly creatures, attuning to and attempting to realize our innate potential at every level. This particular element, for reasons not entirely discernable, appears to embody and promote movement towards what we seek during our life.

——————— Holistic health practices ———————
There are a plethora of different health-enhancing substances and practices available to us in this 'New Age'. We don't have to be expert clinicians or practitioners to have access to the wisdom of the ages that has been 'rediscovered' and reintroduced to us at this time.

These include the many dietary therapies, Chinese medicine and herbs, essential oils, homoeopathy, acupuncture, and crystal and colour healing. We can certainly benefit from the information available on the various techniques and avail ourselves of these therapies when the need arises.

This chapter is an attempt to discuss and bring together, at a common-sense level, some of the many practical ways in which we can significantly enhance our health. The following sections review the current wisdom from orthodox and alternative perspectives concerning factors we can control in our lives, namely what we eat, the amount of exercise we take, and our attitudes to living and relating.

Diet

Of all the factors in our daily life, choosing what we eat is one of the simplest and most effective ways in which we can profoundly influence our health and our attitude towards living. There are many dietary systems. Some of the more well known include macrobiotics, raw food such as the Gerson diet, vegetarianism and the rainbow diet, in which different colour foods are eaten with an awareness of their correspondences to different chakras. Each dietary system usually encompasses a universal philosophy, which goes beyond merely the physical or nutritional basis of foods. Each dietary system embodies truth and wisdom; it is for each of us to choose whatever diet resonates with our being.

During our lifetime, we may go through many changes in our eating practices—after many years of being macrobiotic, we may find that we wish to now incorporate more raw food into our diet. Or, after years of being vegetarian, we may feel comfortable with occasionally eating fish or chicken. Holistic living includes a flexible approach and respect to our growth and needs. What we eat represents more than simply ingesting ingredients; if we take nourishment with awareness and gratitude for its sustenance, then cooking and eating become part of an entire outlook on life that harmonizes with good health.

Irrespective of whichever diet is chosen, there are several common principles which embody good health practice:

1. Choose whole and natural foods and avoid foods and products which have been chemically adulterated. This includes white flour and its products, white rice and packaged convenience foods.
2. Centre the diet on fruits, vegetables, and whole grains,

supplemented with other foods such as fish, poultry, or dairy products.

3. Avoid sugar in all forms, including white and brown sugar and honey.
4. Avoid red meat, eggs, and high fat dairy products.
5. Avoid immuno-depressant substances such as coffee, tea, tobacco, alcohol, and recreational drugs.

Nutritional supplements

In an ideal world with balanced agricultural practices, equal distribution of soil nutrients, no atmospheric or industrial pollution, no radiation, no stress—perhaps sitting atop the rarified atmosphere of the Himalayas—we could, if we led a simple, hard-working life, get all that we needed from our natural diet. And, indeed, an extremely healthy active person may not need to supplement his diet all the time. However, in view of the reality of 'civilized' life, with its pollution, radiation, exhaust fumes, etc., we all could probably benefit from nutritional supplementation from time to time.

Again, as in all things, common-sense and discrimination should be operative words in choosing what supplements to take. There are a myriad of brands available at most health food stores, and stocking up on everything is extremely expensive and results in 'popping' many different capsules every day, which somehow doesn't feel very natural. Accordingly, learn about the various vitamins and minerals and their therapeutic properties,[15,40] and be sensible about your choices. Read the label carefully and don't buy brands with sugar (sucrose, fructose). For a generally healthy person, a multivitamin and mineral tablet may provide an adequate boost to the daily diet; to a person very ill with cancer, AIDS, or a heart condition then it may be advisable to take mega-doses of immuno-enhancing vitamins, minerals, and other extracts.

The most important vitamins and minerals which have known therapeutic properties by virtue of being immuno-enhancers, free radical scavengers, and blood sugar or neuroendocrine modulators include:[5,112]

Vitamins: A, B_6, folic acid, pantothenic acid, C, E.
Minerals: Iron, magnesium, chromium GTF, zinc, selenium, organic germanium.[2,32,34,64,78,79]

In addition to these main supplements, there are many additional health food supplements, such as herbs (ginseng), amino acids and substances such as seaweeds, algae and royal jelly. Again, trust your intuition and discrimination, and read the literature carefully to ensure that these produces will be of benefit to you.

Exercise

Every tradition encourages exercise. From the age-old and contemporary practices of yoga, the oriental martial arts, running, swimming, dancing, skiing, or just plain walking, exercise is good for mind and body. At the mental level, exercise provides a focus for our concentration, and an outlet for expressing pent-up emotions. Exercise when practised as an art can be an exquisite meditation, the ultimate harmonization of mind and body. At the body level, movement benefits the immune system, strengthens the cardiac system, and can increase flexibility, agility, and coordination.

We all know the above, and yet many of us, including myself, do not exercise as optimally as we could. Any programme of exercise, no matter how limited, is of great benefit, because movement can provide one of the greatest sources and inlets to transcendent feelings of calmness, well-being and even ecstasy, for instance 'highs' experienced by long-distance runners.

To make it easy and practical to exercise, determine to spend at least five minutes each morning on some form of exercise. This could entail anything from stretching, yoga, dancing, or walking to the corner and back. A five minute commitment is not too great for any person, yet can produce great benefits.

The most important thing to remember about exercise is that it ought to be enjoyable. Embarking on a fitness routine that is painful or loathsome defeats the entire purpose, which is to enjoy the sheer action of moving the body. Also, choose practices which harmonize with your age, physical condition, and body needs, and which don't torture old injuries or inflict new ones. Be very practical, if the nearest swimming pool is half an hour away and lacks hairdryers, then perhaps swimming should not be your daily exercise.

This is not to deter anyone from following an exercise plan which may be challenging and present difficulties. The advice on choosing simple and short is merely a device to cajole lazy and/or forgetful and unmotivated people from starting to get moving. Any regime which is relished should be indulged in and utilized to full advantage.

Environmental factors

Our environment has a profound effect on the immune system and our entire outlook to living. Environment includes such things as sunlight, which stimulates immune function, radiation, water and air quality. Exposure to sunlight, even five minutes per day (without glasses), is an excellent boost to overall good health. The air we breathe and the water we drink may all contain poisons such as heavy metals and carcinogens, and may severely limit our oxygen supply, so vital for good health. While it is not always possible to vary where we live, it is possible to make choices about the location of our homes based on priorities which support optimum health.

Relating to healthcare: common sense and discrimination

As consumers, we are fortunate indeed to be able to benefit from the knowledge of the orthodox and alternative medical healing professions. However, all too often, due to our unwillingness or inability to take responsibility for our own health, we place ourselves passively into the hands of the 'men in the white coats', expecting them to make us well. This is not to disparage the intent or expertise of the medical profession—modern medicine has achieved much that is invaluable to our lives—rather this is more a comment on our incredible gullibility and the inexplicable faith we have in the mortals in whose care we entrust our bodies. We as health care consumers sometimes surrender our personal power to another person, in whom we invest the authority to heal us.

When we wish to purchase a car, house, stereo, or even a suit or dress, we may spend hours, days, or even longer, researching what is available, discussing the merits of the available products, doubting and being sceptical about what the sales people tell us, trying it, asking the opinions of our friends or lovers, before making a final decision. However, when we take ourselves or our children to the doctor, dentist, or any other practitioner, we are often handed a prescription which is then dispensed at the chemist without us even knowing what has been the diagnosis or what medication has been prescribed. Of course, in theory, these things should be discussed at the time of treatment. However, in the absence of such information, how often do we 'interview' the practitioner about the various kinds of treatments available, what types of side-effects they may have, what will happen if we don't take any medication, etc.

Ultimately, we must decide which treatment we choose, ideally in a co-operative and mutually enriching relationship with the practitioner. The qualities of discrimination, compassion, wisdom, and understanding are all essential ingredients in healing. These should be exercised by the consumer as well as the practitioner. Practitioners have a responsibility to inform and take the utmost care in treating and advising their clients, acting in a manner that serves the highest ideals of their profession. We as consumers have the responsibility to be fully informed and co-operate in an active way with the course of treatment. In this symbiotic fashion, both parties will gain the most.

We are our only healers. Doctors, practitioners, and therapists can and do certainly help us to heal ourselves; however, it is ultimately we who have the illness or condition, and no one can know more about all the details of ourselves than we can. There are definitely times to go to the doctor, take certain medications, undergo surgery, and so on. There are also times when less radical procedures, or perhaps simply relaxing and taking better care of ourselves will work, without having to subject our bodies to drugs, or to needlessly waste our time and that of the practitioner.

Well-being at the emotional and spiritual level

Taking steps to view our life from a holistic perspective has certain inevitable consequences, which all lead to change. First and foremost, the choice to take responsibility for our life puts us squarely in the driver's seat—we control and create our life. We have always been in control, but may not have been aware of it. Additionally, viewing and experiencing life from a holistic perspective means exploring all angles: positive, negative, logical, intuitive, sensible, and irrational. This may be threatening to our beloved sense of security and perhaps result in major explorations outside of narrow career goals, but will ultimately result in heightened awareness, personal development, and spiritual maturity. And, despite our very real and human feelings of inadequacy, hopelessness, and despair, there is nothing more exhilarating and challenging in life than a sense of adventure engendered by knowing that we are our own potential instrument of change.

As we progress further along the path of self-discovery, there comes a point at which we glimpse some fragment of who we are, and perhaps why we are here or what our true inner essence is. In my view, if life has any 'purpose', it is to enable us to realize the fulfilment of our truest potential. This is not said from an outwardly ambitious viewpoint of money and career, but rather from a perspective of finding deep enriching satisfaction in our lives.

Each of us is unique, and we are always moving towards the attainment of our individual paths. Within each of us is our own inner wisdom, intuition, and knowing which can guide us in our individual quests toward self-realization and fulfilment. Dr Asai found deep spiritual satisfaction and realized many insights with his discoveries and development of organic germanium. For each of us, this search and discovery will take many different forms. Only our inner voices can guide us to the treasures contained within. Good health and life-enhancing practices are invaluable assets which we should strive to maintain in order to arrive at our destinies.

Fun and self acceptance

In conclusion and above all else, fun and enjoyment is of principal importance. 'Seriousness' can become a number one disease. Fun means giving yourself permission to be yourself—not some submissive robot. We can all benefit from being in touch with our mischievous side, remembering a few good jokes, not being so boringly predictable. For, no matter how well we plan things, or how careful we may be, we never know for certain for how long we will be around. The best recipe for a happy life is to enjoy every moment to its fullest. To relish everything, the bad, the sad, along with the happy, to experiment and not be afraid of making mistakes, because there are no such things as mistakes, only lessons.

References

1. Arimori, S. Watanabe, K. Yoshida, M. and Nagao, T. 'Effect of Ge-132 as immunomodulator'. In *Immunomodulation by Microbial Products and Related Synthetic Compounds. Int. Symp.*, Osaka, July 27–29, 1981. Yamamura and Kotani (eds.), Exerpta Medica, 498–500. 1982.

2. Asai, K. *Miracle Cure: Organic Germanium*, Japan Publications Inc. 1980.

3. Aso, H., Suzuki, F., Yamaguchi, T., Hayashi, Y., Ebina, T., and Ishida, N. 'Induction of interferon and activation of NK cells and macrophages in mice by oral administration of Ge-132, an organic germanium compound'. *Microbiol. Immunol.*, **29**, 65–74. 1985.

4. Badger, A.M., Mirabelli, O.K. and DiMartino, M., 'Generation of suppressor cells in normal rats by treatment with Spiro-germanium, a novel heterocyclic anticancer drug'. *Immunopharmacology*, **10**, 201–7. 1985.

5. Badgley, L. *Healing Aids Naturally. Natural Therapies for the Immune System*, Human Energy Press, 1986.

6. Bolen, J.S., *Goddesses in Every Woman. A New Pscyhology of Women*, Harper Colofon, 1984.

7. Bonewitz, R., *Cosmic Crystals. Crystal Consciousness and the New Age*, Thorsons, 1983.

8. Boros, L., Tsiatis, A.A., Neiman, R.S., Mann, R.B. and Glick

J.H., 'Phase II Eastern Co-operative Oncology Group Study of Spirogermanium in previously treated lymphoma'. *Cancer Treat. Rep.*, **70**, 917–8. 1986.

9. Bradford. W., Culbert, M.L. and Allen, H.W., *International Protocols for Individualized, Integrated Metabolic Programs in Cancer Management.* Robert W. Bradford Foundation, 1983.

10. Bradford, R.W., Allen, H.W., and Culbert, M.L., *Oxidology. The Study of Reactive Oxygen Toxic Species (ROTS) and their Metabolism in Health and Disease.* Robert W. Bradford Foundation, 1985.

11. Brenner, D.E., Rosenshein, N.E., Dillon M., Jones H.W., Forastiere, A., Tipping, S., Burnett, L.S., Greco, F.A., and Wiernick, P.H., Phase II study of Spirogermanium in patients with advanced carcinoma of the cervix, *Cancer Treat. Rep.*, **69**, 457–8. 1985.

12. Brenner, D.E., Jones, H.W., Rosenshein, N.B., Forastiere, A., Dillon, M., Grumbine, F., Tipping, S., Burnett, L., Greco, F.A. and Wiernik, P.H., 'Phase II evaluation of spirogermanium in advanced ovarian carcinoma'. *Cancer Treat. Rep.* **67**, 193–4. 1983.

13. Brodbeck, J., Germanium in biological systems'. In *1st Int. Conf. on Germanium*, Hanover, Oct. 1984. Lekim and Samochowiec (eds.) Semmelweis-Verlag. 1985.

14. Colbin, A. *The Book of Whole Meals*, Ballantine Books, 1979. 1983

15. Davies, S., *Nutritional Medicine*, Pan Books, 1987.

16. Davidson, J.H., *Radiation: What it is, how it affects us and what we can do about it*, C.W. Daniel, 1986.

17. De Vries, J., *Do Miracles Exist*, Mainstream Publishing, 1986.

18. De Vries, J., *Multiple Sclerosis*, Mainstream Publishing, 1985.

19. Dexeus, F.H., Logothetis, C., Samuels, M.L. and Hossan, B., 'Phase II study of Spirogermanium in metastatic prostate cancer'. *Cancer Treat Rep.*, **70**(9), 1129–30, 1986.

20. Dhingra, H.M., Unsawaski, T., Chiuten, D.F., Murphy, W.K., Holoye, P.Y., Spitzer, G. and Valdivieso, M., 'Phase II study of spirogermanium in advanced (extensive) non-small cell lung cancer'. *Cancer Treat. Rep.*, **70**, 673–4, 1986.

21. DiMartino, M.J., Lee, J.C., Badger, A.M., Muirhead, K.A.,

Mirabelli, C.K. and Hanna, N., Antiarthritic and immuno-regulatory activity of spirogermanium'. *J. Pharmacol. Exp. Ther.*, **236**, 103–10, 1986.

22. Dluzniewski, A., Gastol-Lewinska, L., Buczynska, B. and Monicqewski, A., 'Teratogenic effects of Sanumgerman in rats'. In *1st Int. Conf. on Germanium,* Hanover, October 1984, Lekim and Samochowiec (eds.), Semmelweis-Verlag, 1985.

23. Diekmann, K., Widderlich, Widderich, M., and Wilgenbus, U., Doctoral Dissertations, Institute fur Physiologische Chemi der Tierarztlichen Hochschule, Hanover. 1985–86.

24. Eisenhauer, E., Quirt, I., Connors, J.M. Maroun, J. and Skillings, J., 'A Phase II study of Spirogermanium as second line therapy in patients with poor prognosis lymphoma', An NCI Canada Clinical Trials Group Study, *Invest New Drugs*, **3**, 307–10, 1985

25. Eisenhauer, E., Kerr, I., Bodurtha, A., Iscoe, N., McCullock, P., Pritchard, K. and Quirt, I., 'A Phase II study of Spirogermanium in patients with metastatic malignant melanoma, An NCI Canada Clinical Trials Group Study, *Invest New Drugs*, **3**, 303–5. 1985.

26. Falkson, G., and Falkson, H.C., 'Phase II trial of Spirogermanium for treatment of advanced breast cancer', *Cancer Treat. Rep.*, **67**, 189–90, 1983.

27. Gallo, R.C., 'The AIDS virus'. *Scientific American*, **256** (January) 38–61, 1987.

28. Gallo R.C., 'The first human retrovirus'. *Scientific American*, **255** (December), 78–88, 1986.

29. *Ge-132 Outline*, Asai Germanium Res. Inst., 1984.

30. Gieldanowski, J., 'The Influence of Sanumgerman on the induction of spontaneous leukemia and the activity of killer cells (NK)', 1986 and 'Mutagenicity Tests on Sanumgerman, Polish Academy of Sciences, Ludwik Hirszfeld Institute of Immunology and Experimental Therapy, 1987.

31. Goodman, S., 'Organic germanium – powerful healer'. *J. Alt. & Comp. Med.*, **4**, 34–52, 1987.

32. Goodman, S., 'Between physics and biology'. *J. Alt. & Comp. Med.*, **5** (9), 21–2. 1987.

33. Goodman, S. *Therapeutic Effects of Organic Germanium. Medical Hypothesis*, In Press, 1987.

34. Graham, J. and Odent, M., *The Z Factor. How Zinc is Vital to Your Health*, Thorsons, 1986.

35. Grzybek, J., 'Biological activity of Sanumgerman in allium test'. In *1st Int. Conf. on Germanium*, Hanover, October 1984. Lekim and Samochowiec (eds.) Semmelweis-Verlag, 1985.

36. Hachisu, M., Takahashi, H., Koeda, T. and Sekizawa, Y., 'Analgesic effect of novel organogermanium compound, Ge-132'. *J. Pharmacobiodyn*, **6**, 814–20, 1983.

37. Harisch, G., 'Glutathione and glutathione-dependent enzymes of the rat liver after different doses of Sanumgerman'. In *1st Int. Conf. on Germanium*, Hanover, October 1984, Lekim and Samochowiec (eds.) Semmelweis-Verlag. 1985.

38. Hill, B.T., Bellamy, A.S., Metcalfe, S., Hepburn, P.J., Masters, J.R., and Whelan, R.D., 'Idenfication of synergistic combinations of Spirogermanium with 5-fluorouracil or cisplatin using a range of human tumour cell lines *in vitro*'. *Invest New Drugs*, **2**, 29–33, 1984.

39. Hill, B., Whatley, S.A., Bellamy, A.S., Jenkins, L.H. and Whelan, R.D.H., 'Cytotoxic effects and biological activities of NSC-192965; Spirogermanium *in vitro*'. *Cancer Res.*, **42**, 2852–6, 1982.

40. Holford, P., *The Whole Health Guide to Elemental Health and Vitamin Vitality*, Thorsons, 1983.

41. Hueper, W.C., 'Effects of overdoses of germanium dioxide upon the blood and tissues of rabbits'. *Am. J. Med. Sciences*, **181**, 820–30, 1931.

42. Ingeborg, S., 'Germanium—from the general practice—for the general practice'. In *1st Int. Conf. on Germanium*, Hanover, October 1984, Lekim and Samochowiec (eds.), Semmelweis-Verlag. 1985.

43. Ishida, N., Satoh, H., Suzuki, F. and Miyao, K., *Organo-germanium Induction of Interferon Production*, United States Patent No. 4, 473, 581, 1984.

44. Kada, T., Mochizuki, H., and Miyao, K., 'Antimutagenic effects of germanium oxide on Trp-P-2 induced frameshift mutations in *Salmonella typhimurium* TA98 and TA 1538', *Mutation Research*, **125**, 145–51. 1984.

45. Kamen, B., Germanium—A New Approach to Immunity, Nutrition Encounter Inc., Larkspur, California, 1987.

46. Kavanagh, J.J., Saul, P.B., Copeland, L.J., Gershenson, D.M. and Krakoff, I.H., 'Continuous infusion spirogermanium for the treatment of refractory carcinoma of the ovary: a phase II trial', *Cancer Treat. Rep.*, **69**, 139–40, 1985.

47. Kidd, P.M., *Networking and Consulting Services on Germanium*, GINA, 1987.

48. Kidd, S., 'Germanium-132 (Ge-132) Homeostatic normalizer and immunostimulant. A review of its preventive and therapeutic efficacy', *Int. Clin. Nutr. Rev.* **7**(1), 1987.

49. Kidd, P.M., *Therapeutic Potentialities for Ge-132*, GINA, 1987.

50. Kleinrok, Z., Lekim, D., Jagiello-Wojtowicz, E. and Chodkowska, A., 'Central action of sanumgerman in mice', *Pol. J. Pharmacol. Pharm.*, **38**, 299·307, 1986.

51. Kleinrock, Z., Jagiello-Wojtowicz, E. and Chodkowska, A., In *1st Int. Conf. on Germanium*, Hanover, October 1984, Lekim and Samochowiec (eds.), Semmelweis-Verlag, 1985.

52. Kobayshi, H., Komuro, T. and Furue, H., 'Effect of combination immunochemotherapy with an organo-germanium compound, Ge-132, and antitumor agents on C57BL/6 mice bearing Lewis lung carcinoma (3LL)'. *Gan-To-Kagaku-Ryoho*, **13**, 2588–93, 1986.

53. Kohlmunzer, S., 'The allium test as a tool in search for potential oncostatics, In *1st Int. Conf. on Germanium*, Hanover, October 1984, Lekim and Samochowiec (eds.) Semmelweis-Verlag, 1985.

54. Kokoschinegg, P., and Kokoshinegg, M., 'Biophysical results with germanium and Sanumgerman—preliminary experiences', In *1st Int. Conf. on Germanium*, Hanover, October 1984, Lekim and Samochowiec (eds.) Semmelweis-Verlag, 1985.

55. Komuro, T., Kakimoto, N., Katayama, T. and Hazato, T., 'Inhibitory effects of Ge-132 (carboxyethyl germanium sesquioxide derivatives on enkephalin-degrading enzymes', *Biotechnol. Appl. Biochem.*, **8**, 379–86, 1986.

56. Kuebler, J.P., Tormey D.C., Harper, G. R., Chang, Y.C., Khandekar, J.D. and Falkson, G., 'Phase II study of Spiro-germanium in advanced breast cancer', *Cancer Treat, Rep.*, **68**, 1515–16, 1984.

57. Kumano, N. Ishikawa, T., Koinumar, S., Kikumoto, T., Suzuki,

S., Nakai, Y. and Konno K., 'Antitumour effect of the organogermanium compound Ge-132 on the Lewis lung carcinoma (3LL) in C57BL/6 (B6) mice', *Tohoku J. Exp. Med.*, **146**, 97–104, 1985..

58. Lekim, D., and Kehlbeck, H., 'The biological activity of germanium, In *1st Int. Conf. on Germanium*, Hanover, October 1984, Lekim and Samochowiec (eds.) Semmelweis-Verlag, 1985.

59. Lekim, D., Samochowiec, L. and Gieldanowski, J., 'Oncostatic properties of Sanumgerman. In *1st Int. Conf. on Germanium*, Hanover, October 1984, Lekim and Samochowiec (eds.) Semmelweis-Verlag, 1985.

60. Lekim, D., Samochowiec, L. and Gieldanowski, J., 'Results of studies on antineoplastic activity of Sanumgerman preparation', In *1st Int. Conf. on Germanium*, Hanover, October 1984, Lekim and Samochowiec (eds.) Semmelweis-Verlag, 1985.

61. Levan, A., 'The effects of colchicine on root mitoses in allium. *Hereditas*, **24**, 471, 1938.

62. Levine, S.A., and Kidd, P.M., 'Oxygen nutrition for super health'. *J. Orthomolecular Medicine*, **1** (3), 145–8, 1986.

63. Levine, S. and Huntington, K., 'Organic germanium: restoring health through increased oxygenation', *Total Health*, **18**, 1986.

64. Lewis, A., *Selenium: The essential trace element you might not be getting enough of*, Thorsons, 1983.

65. Liem, S.H., 'The influence of Sanumgerman on the oxygen partial pressure of the oxygen multi-step process'. In *1st Int. Conf. on Germanium*, Hanover, October 1984, Lekim and Samochowiec (eds.) Semmelweis-Verlag, 1985.

66. Martin, S., 'Germanium: could it be the cure?' *Here's Health*, April 1987, pp 12–14.

67. Melnik, S.I., Bakhmedova, A.A., Nedorezova, T.P., Iartseva, I.V. and Zhukova, O.S., 'Synthesis of anomeric 5-trimethylgermyl-2-deoxyuridines and study of their antiviral and cytotoxic properties'. *Bioorg Khim.*, **11**, 1248–52, 1985.

68. Mino, Y., Ota, N., Sakao, S. and Shimomura, S., 'Determination of germanium in medicinal plants by atomic absorption spectrometry with electrothermal atomization'. *Chem. Phar. Bull.*, **28** (9), 2687–91, 1980.

69. Miyao, K., Onishi, T., Asai, K., Tomizawa, S. and Suzuki, F., 'Toxicology and Phase I studies on a novel organogermanium compound, Ge-132'. *Current Chemother. & Inf. Dis. Proc. 11th ICC and 19th ICAAC Amer. Soc. Micro.*, 80–2, 1980.

70. Mizushima, M., Satoh, H. and Miyao, K., 'Some pharmacological and clinical aspects of a novel organic germanium compound Ge-132'. In *1st Int. Conf. on Germanium*, Hanover, October 1984, Lekim and Samochowiec (eds.) Semmelweis-Verlag, 1985.

71. Mizushima, Y., Shoji, Y. and Kaneko, K., 'Restoration of impaired immunoresponse by germanium in mice'. *Int. Arch. Allergy Appl. Immunol.* **63**, 338–9, 1980.

72. Mochizuki, H. and Kada, T., 'Antimutagenic effect of Ge-132 on gamma-ray-induced mutations in *E. coli* B/r WP2 trp-'. *Int. J. Radiat. Biol.*, **42**(6), 653–9, 1982.

73. Mrema, J.E., Slavik, M. and Davis, J., 'Spirogermanium: a new drug with antimalarial activity against chloroquine-resistant *Plasmodium falciparum*, *Int. J. Clin. Pharmacol. Ther. Tox.*, **4**, 167–71, 1983.

74. Nagata, N., Yoneyama, T., Yanagida, K., Ushio, K., Yanagihara, S., Matsubara, O. and Eishi, Y., 'Accumulation of germanium in the tissues of a long-term user of germanium preparation died of acture renal failure, *J. Toxicol. Sci.*, **10**, 333–41, 1985.

75. *New Scientist*. ... or can the body protect itself? 18 December, 7, 1986.

76. Paetz, G., 'Case study: adenocarcinoma with liver metastases'. In *1st Int. Conf. on Germanium*, Hanover, October 1984, Lekim and Samochowiec (eds.) Semmelweis-Verlag, 1985.

77. Paetz, G., 'A therapy with new dimensions: Sanumgerman'. *Raum and Zeit*. 24/86, 12–13, 1986.

78. Passwater, R.A., *Selenium as Food and Medicine*, Keats Publishing, 1980.

79. Passwater, R.A., *GTF Chromium*, Keats Publishing, 1982.

80. Pfeiffer, C.C., *Mental illness and Schizophrenia. The Nutrition Connection*, Thorsons, 1987.

81. Pinnameneni, K., Yap, H.Y., Kegha, S.S., Blumenschein, G. R. and Bodey, G. P., 'Phase II study of Spirogermanium in the treatment of metastic breast cancer, *Cancer Treat. Rep.*, **68**,

1197–8, 1984.

82. Rice, L.M., Wheeler. W.J., and Geschickter, C.F. 'Synthesis of 4, 4-diakyl-4-4 germacyclohexanone and 8,8-diakyl-8-germanspiro 8 (4.5) decanes', *J. Heterocyclic Chem.*, **11**, 1041–7, 1984.

83. Rosenfield, G. and Wallace, E.J., 'Studies of the acute and chronic toxicity of germanium', *Arch. Indus. Hygiene Occ. Med.*, **8**, 466–79, 1953.

84. Samochowiec, L., 'Experience with Sanumgerman in Poland and Germany'. In *1st Int. Conf. on Germanium*, Hanover, October 1984, Lekim and Samochowiec (eds.) Semmelweis-Verlag, 1985.

85. Samochowiec, L. and Wojcicki, J., 'Basic pharmacological properties of Sanumgerman'. In *1st Int. Conf. on Germanium*, Hanover, October 1984, Lekim and Samochowiec (eds.) Semmelweis-Verlag, 1985.

86. Sato, I., Yuan, B.D. Nishimura, T. and Tanaka, N., 'Inhibition of tumor growth and metastasis in association with modification of immune response by novel organic germanium compounds'. *J. Biol. Response Mod.*, **4**, 159–68, 1985.

87. Schein, P.S., 'The clinical pharmacology of Spirogermanium, a unique anti cancer agent'. In *1st Int. Conf. on Germanium*, Hanover, October 1984, Lekim and Samochowiec (eds.) Semmelweis-Verlag, 1985.

88. Schein, P.S., Slavik, M. Smythe, T., Hoth D, Smith, F., Macdonald, J.S. and Woolley, P.V., 'Phase I clinical trial of Spirogermanium', *Cancer Treat. Rep.*, **64**, 1051–6, 1980.

89. Schroeder, H.A., Kanisawa, M., Frost, D.V. and Mitchener, M., 'Germanium, tin and arsenic in rats: effects on growth, survival, pathological lesions and life span', *J. Nutrition*, **96**, 37–45, 1968.

90. Schroeder, H.A. and Balassa, J.J., 'Arsenic, germanium, tin and vanadium in mice. Effects on growth, survival and tissue levels, *J. Nutrition*, **92** 245–52, 1967.

91. Schroeder, H.A. and Balassa, J.J., 'Abnormal trace metals in man: germanium'. *J. Chron. Dis.*, **20**, 211–24, 1967.

92. Schuitemaker, G.E., 'Germanium: a mineral of great promise. *OrthoMoleculair*, No. 3, 1987.

93. Schulman, P., David, R.B., Rafla, S., Green M. and Henderson, E., 'Phase II trial of Spirogermanium in advanced renal cell carcinoma: a Cancer and Leukemia Group B study', *Cancer Treat. Rep.*, **68**, 1305–6, 1984.

94. Sijpesteijn, A.K., Rijkins, F. and Van der Kerk, G.J.M., 'Antimicrobial activity of trialkylgermanium acetates and the influence of the medium', *Antonie van Loeuwenhock*, **30**, 113–20, 1964.

95. Soloman, G.F., 'The emerging field of psychoneuro-immunology, with a special note on AIDS'. *Advances, Institute for the Advancement of Health*, **2**(1), 6–19, 1985.

96. Stortebecker, P., *Mercury Poisoning from Dental Amalgam—a Hazard to Human Brain*, Stortebecker Foundation for Research, 1985.

97. Suzuki, T., Ishikawa, S., Motoyama T. and Oboshi, S., 'Suppression and acceleration of experimental amyloidosis in mouse model'. *Acta Pathol. Japan*, **30**(4), 557–64, 1980.

98. Suzuki, F., 'Antitumour activity of Ge-132, a new organogermanium compound, in mice is expressed through the functions of macrophages and T lympocytes', *Gan-To Kagaku Rhoho*, **12**, 1445–52, 1985.

99. Suzuki, F., 'Suppression of tumor growth by peritoneal macrophages isolated from mice treated with carboxyethyl-germanium sesquioxide (Ge-132)'. *Gan To Kagaku Ryoho*, **12**, 2122–8, 1985.

100. Suzuki, F., 'Ability of sera from mice treated with Ge-132, an organo-germanium compound, to inhibit experimental murine asictes tumors', *Gan To Kagaku Ryoho*, **12**, 2314–21, 1985.

101. Suzuki, G. and Pollard, R.B., 'Prevention of suppressed interferon gamma production in thermally injured mice by administration of a novel organogermanium compound, Ge-132', *J. Interferon Res.*, **4**, 223–33, 1984.

102. Suzuki, F., Brutkiewicz, R.R., and Pollard, R.B., 'Importance of T-cells and macrophages in the antitumour activity of carboxyethylgermanium sesquioxide (Ge-132)', *Anticancer Res.*, **5**, 479–83, 1985.

103. Suzuki, F., Brutkiewicz, R.R., and Pollard, R.B., 'Co-operation of lymphokine(s) and macrophages in expression of antitumor activity of carboxyethylgermanium sesquioxide (Ge-132)'.

Anticancer Res., **6**, 177–82, 1986.

104. Takashima R. and Mitsui, Y., 'Germanium as a stabilizer of cysteine eye drop', In *Immunomodulation by Microb. Products and related synthetic compounds. Int. Symp.* Osaka, 27–29 July 1981, Yamamura & Kotani (eds.) Exerpta Medica, 498–500, 1982.

105. Tanaka, N, Ohida, J. Ono, M, Yoshiwara, H, Beika, T., Terasawa, A., Yamada, J., Morioka, S., Mannami, T. and Orita, K., 'Augmentation of NK activity in peripheral blood lymphocyte in cancer patients by intermittent Ge-132 administration. *Gan To Kagaku Ryoho*, **11**, 1303–6, 1984.

106. Trope, C., Mattsson, W., Gynning, I., Johnson, J.E., Sigurdsson, K. and Orbert, B., 'Phase II study of Spirogermanium in advanced ovarian malignancy', *Cancer Treat. Rep.*, **65**, 119–20, 1981.

107. Tsutsui, M., Kakimoto, M., Axtell, D.D., Oikawa, H. and Asai, K., 'Crystal structure of carboxyethylgermanium sesquioxide', *J. Amer. Chem. Soc.*, **98**(25), 8287–9, 1976.

108. Vogelzang, N.J., Gesme, D.H. and Kennedy, B.J., 'A phase II study of Spirogermanium in advanced human malignancy, *Am. J. Clin. Oncol.*, **8**, 341–4, 1985.

109. Walker, C.M., Moody, D.J., Stites, D. P. and Levy, J.A., 'CDB lymphocytes can control HIV infection *in vitro* by suppressing virus replication', *Science*, **234**, 1563–6, 1986.

110. Watschinger, G., 'Germanium, an extraordinary trace element in biological systems', In *1st Int. Conf. on Germanium*, Hanover, October 1984, Lekim and Samochowiec (eds.) Semmelweis-Verlag, 1985.

111. Webb, T. and Lang, T., *Food Irradiation: The Facts*, Thorsons, 1987.

112. Weiner, M.A., *Maximum Immunity: How to fortify your natural defences against cancer, AIDS, arthritis, allergies and other immune deficiency diseases.* Gateway Books, 1986.

113. Whipple, G.H. and Robscheit-Robbins, F.S., 'Blood regeneration in severe anemia', *Am. J. Physiol.*, **72**, 419–30, 1925.

114. Wodinsky, *et al.*, *Screening Data Summaries.* Drug Research & Dev. Program, Division of Cancer Treatment, National Cancer Institute, Bethesda, MA, 1977.

115. Woodman, M., *The Pregnant Virgin. A Process of Psychological Transformation*, Webcom, 1985.

116. Woolley, P.V., Ahlgren, J.D., Byrne, P.J., Priego, V.M. and Schein, P.S., 'A phase I trial of Spirogermanium administered on a continuous infusion schedule, *Invest New Drugs*, **2**, 305–9, 1984.

117. Yang S.J. and Rafla, S., 'Effect of Spirogermanium on V79 Chinese hamster cells', *Am. J. Clin. Oncol.*, **6**, 331–7, 1983.

118. Ziff, S., *The Toxic Time Bomb*, Thorsons, 1985.

119. Zoubek, E., 'The Sanumgerman therapy in biological medicine', In *1st Int. Conf. on Germanium*, Hanover, October 1984, Lekim and Samochowiec (eds.) Semmelweis-Verlag, 1985.

Index